T0313894

KAREN BIRMINGHAM

# PIONEERING ETHICS IN A LONGITUDINAL STUDY

The early development of the ALSPAC
Ethics and Law Committee

FOREWORD BY JEAN GOLDING

POLICY PRESS SHORTS RESEARCH

First published in Great Britain in 2018 by

Policy Press
University of Bristol
1-9 Old Park Hill
Bristol
BS2 8BB
UK
t: +44 (0)117 954 5940
pp-info@bristol.ac.uk
www.policypress.co.uk

North America office:
Policy Press
c/o The University of Chicago Press
1427 East 60th Street
Chicago, IL 60637, USA
t: +1 773 702 7700
f: +1 773 702 9756
sales@press.uchicago.edu
www.press.uchicago.edu

British Library Cataloguing in Publication Data
A catalogue record for this book is available from the British Library.

Library of Congress Cataloging-in-Publication Data
A catalog record for this book has been requested.

ISBN 978-1-4473-4038-6  (hardback)
ISBN 978-1-4473-4039-3  (ePub)
ISBN 978-1-4473-4040-9  (Mobi)
ISBN 978-1-4473-4042-3  (OA PDF)

Cover design by Policy Press
Front cover: image kindly supplied by Shutterstock
Printed and bound in Great Britain by CPI Group (UK) Ltd,
Croydon, CR0 4YY
Policy Press uses environmentally responsible print partners

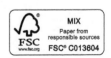

# Contents

# List of figures and photographs

## Figures

## Photographs

# List of abbreviations

| | |
|---|---|
| AELC | ALSPAC Ethics and Law Committee |
| ALEC | ALSPAC Ethics and Law Committee |
| ALSPAC | Avon Longitudinal Study of Parents and Children, previously known as Avon Longitudinal Study of Pregnancy and Childhood |
| BCC | Bristol City Council |
| BPA | British Paediatric Association |
| CiF | Children in Focus: research clinics for 10% subsample of ALSPAC |
| Co90s | Children of the 90s (ALSPAC as known by the Study participants) |
| COREC | Central Office for Research Ethics Committees |
| DfES | Department for Education and Skills |
| ELSPAC | European Study of Pregnancy and Childhood |
| EPEG | Ethical Protection in Epidemiological Genetic Research: Participants' Perspective |
| ERC | Ethics of Research Committee |
| F@7 (8, 9, 10, 11) | ALSPAC research clinics for participants at age seven, eight, nine, 10 and 11 |

| | |
|---|---|
| Focus@7 (8, 9, 10, 11) | ALSPAC research clinics for participants at age seven, eight, nine, 10 and 11 |
| Focus at 7 (8, 9, 10, 11) | ALSPAC research clinics for participants at age seven, eight, nine, 10 and 11 |
| HGC | Human Genetics Commission |
| HV | Health Visitor |
| IRB | Institutional Review Board |
| LREC | Local Research Ethics Committee (NHS) |
| MRC | Medical Research Council |
| NHS | National Health Service |
| NSC | National Screening Committee |
| ONS | Office for National Statistics |
| PIAG | Patient Information Advisory Group |
| PIS | Participant Information Sheet |
| RCP | Royal College of Physicians |
| REC | Research Ethics Committee (NHS) |
| Teen Focus 1 | ALSPAC research clinic for participants at age 12 |
| Teen Focus 1 *fasttrack* | Briefer ALSPAC research clinic for participants at age 12 |
| Teen Focus 2 | ALSPAC research clinic for participants at age 13 |
| Teen Focus 3 | ALSPAC research clinic for participants at age 15 |
| Teen Focus 4 | ALSPAC research clinic for participants at age 17 |
| TF1 | ALSPAC research clinic for participants at age 12 |
| TF1*ft* | Briefer ALSPAC research clinic for participants at age 12 |
| TF2 | ALSPAC research clinic for participants at age 13 |

| | |
|---|---|
| TF3 | ALSPAC research clinic for participants at age 15 |
| TF4 | ALSPAC research clinic for participants at age 17 |
| UOB | University of Bristol |
| WHO | World Health Organisation |
| WT | Wellcome Trust |

# Authors and contributors, with current positions

## Professor Richard Ashcroft

- Professor of Bioethics, Queen Mary, University of London
- Member of the ALSPAC Ethics and Law Committee: September 1998 to March 2000
- ALSPAC collaborator and principle investigator on Wellcome-funded qualitative study: Ethical Protection in Epidemiological Genetic Research: Participants Perspectives (EPEG)
- Interviewed in Queen Mary, London, February 2013

## Miss Karen Birmingham

- Research Fellow, Centre for Child & Adolescent Health, University of Bristol
- Secretary of the ALSPAC Ethics and Law Committee: December 1999 to April 2013

## Dr Tim Chambers

- Consultant Paediatrician, retired
- Founding member of the ALSPAC Ethics and Law Committee: May 1990 to June 1997
- Interviewed in Barley House (University of Bristol), February 2013

## Professor Michael Furmston

- Professor of Law, Sunway University, Malaysia
- Emeritus Professor of Law, University of Bristol
- Chair of the ALSPAC Ethics and Law Committee from its initial meeting in April 1990 to September 2006
- Interviewed in his UK home in Bridgwater, Somerset, December 2012

## Professor Jean Golding

- Emeritus Professor of Paediatric & Perinatal Epidemiology, University of Bristol
- As Director of ALSPAC, in attendance at every ALSPAC Ethics and Law Committee meeting, almost without exception, from initial meeting in April 1990 to retirement in July 2005
- Interviewed at home in Clevedon, Somerset, December 2012

## Dr David Jewell

- General Practitioner, Bristol, retired
- Member of the ALSPAC Ethics and Law Committee: June 2000 to September 2013
- Chair of the ALSPAC Ethics and Law Committee: January 2010 to September 2013
- Interviewed in Barley House (University of Bristol), December 2012

## Dr Ian Lister Cheese

- Senior Medical Officer, Department of Health, retired
- Founding member of the ALSPAC Ethics and Law Committee: April 1990 to July 2000
- Interviewed at home in Wantage, Oxfordshire, April 2013

## Mrs Elizabeth Mumford

- Teaching Fellow in Law, University of Bristol
- Secretary of the ALSPAC Ethics and Law Committee from initial meeting in April 1990 to December 1999
- Continued as member of the ALSPAC Ethics and Law Committee until October 2011
- Interviewed in Barley House (University of Bristol), February 2013

## Professor Marcus Pembrey

- Emeritus Professor of Paediatric Genetics, University College, London
- ALSPAC Director of Genetics, not a member of the ALSPAC Ethics and Law Committee, but advised on genetic issues
- Interviewed at home in Mersea Island, Essex, February 2013

## Professor Gordon Stirrat

- Emeritus Professor of Obstetrics and Gynaecology, University of Bristol
- Founding member of the ALSPAC Ethics and Law Committee with a two-year break in membership when Dean of Faculty of Medicine
- Chair of the ALSPAC Ethics and Law Committee from September 2006 to December 2009
- Interviewed in Barley House (University of Bristol), February 2013

# Acknowledgements

My thanks to:

- Jean Golding, none of which could have been achieved without her, not only for establishing and directing ALSPAC while maintaining an unwavering commitment to the ethical underpinning of the Study, but also for her constant and enthusiastic personal support, enabling the ALSPAC Ethics Archive to be created and this book to be written.
- Michael Furmston for his inspiring chairmanship of the Committee for so many years and the other members of the Committee from whom I have learnt so much.
- All those who agreed to be interviewed and have been extensively quoted throughout.
- Hugh Barnes, Richard Jones and Elizabeth Mumford for their suggestions and perspective.
- Linda Wilson, who spent many hours scanning the documents to create the ALSPAC Ethics Archive and Jill Kelly, who created some order from the initial mass of archival documents.
- The Leverhulme Trust, which financed the process of creating the ALSPAC Ethics Archive.
- The Brocher Foundation, which awarded me a visiting researcher post during September and October 2012, providing the facilities and peace and quiet to enable me to begin writing the book.

- The University of Bristol Alumni, which financed the brief oral histories through the Dean of the Faculty of Medicine and Dentistry Award.
- The Wellcome Trust, which financed both scoping (Grant ref 096605/Z/11/Z) and cataloguing (Grant ref 106783/Z/15/Z) of the ALSPAC Administrative Archive, including the ALSPAC Ethics Archive, by the University of Bristol Library Special Collections. The Wellcome Trust also, alongside the UK Medical Research Council (Grant ref: 102215/2/13/2) and the University of Bristol, continue to provide core support for ALSPAC.
- All the families who took part in the Study, the midwives for their help in recruiting them and the whole ALSPAC team, which includes interviewers, computer and laboratory technicians, clerical workers, research scientists, volunteers, managers, receptionists, and nurses.

The current ALSPAC Executive Committee has read and is happy to endorse this book.

# Foreword

It was a privilege to have the opportunity of initiating and directing the Avon Longitudinal Study of Parents and Children (ALSPAC), even though when times were particularly tough, it seemed like a self-imposed treadmill. Such times were more to do with raising enough money to keep the Study going rather than the Study itself, which was exciting and rewarding in itself. As will be seen from this book, the Study was pioneering in many ways, and the Ethics Committee was vital in guiding it. It was the late, and much missed, Professor David Baum whose idea it was to have such a committee, and it was he who had the foresight to suggest Michael Furmston as the Chair. Both ideas were inspirational. As will be seen from this volume, the way in which the Committee worked derived largely from that choice of Chair.

To put the Study in context, Britain was famous for its longitudinal birth cohort studies, especially the three previous national surveys of births in 1946, 1958 and 1970. Having worked on the last two of these, I was aware of the advantages and defects in such studies – the advantages being that they were population-based, with high response rates, the disadvantages being that they lacked the depth that could have been found with more frequent contacts and observations. I therefore developed a design in the 1980s based on the latest (at that time) ideas as to what was known and what was not known. Surprisingly little was known about the ways in which different features of the environment influenced the health and development of the child but evidence from the study of malformations and childhood leukaemia showed that pregnancy was an important time, and that factors such as medications (for example thalidomide) and infections (for example rubella) could have profound effects. What was not known was how such features might have more subtle influences that would not be apparent until mid-childhood or later. Added to this was the possibility that there were subtle genetic effects that may have direct influences on development, or that may only have influences in the presence of specific environments.

Given this background, it was obvious that the design of the Study should be to collect as much information as possible on the environment of the parents up until the time of pregnancy and to continue to monitor this, and that of the child, thereafter. The obvious time to start collecting data was as early in pregnancy as possible. This was the first way in which ALSPAC differed from other British birth cohorts. The second unique feature concerned the decision to collect data using self-completion questionnaires rather than by interview; this we considered important for two reasons – it was cheaper but, more importantly, the participants would have the advantage of having time to find answers (such as by looking at diaries or asking a family member) and thus provide more accurate information. Third, the Study was innovative in collecting biological samples as a means of identifying exposures to chemicals, as well as providing the opportunity to extract DNA and assay levels of hormones and metabolites of various sorts. Fourth, and equally importantly, it was innovative in its approach to ethics and the creation of its own ethics committee.

None of the previous cohorts had felt the need to consider the ethics of what they were doing until the mid-1980s, when Neville Butler decided that the plans for the medical examination included in the 16-year-old sweep of the 1970 birth cohort should be considered by a Local Research Ethics Committee. However, it was unique to have an ethics committee attached to a Study. This proved to be a major asset to the Study and to me in particular.

As Director of the Study, I was acutely aware of the responsibilities entailed. My husband had been in the army during the Second World War and was particularly keen on asking "Where does the buck stop?". Obviously, it stopped with me. Any breach of confidentiality, any error in the science and any difficulty with the financial probity of the Study would ultimately fall on me. As Karen has documented so well in this volume, as time went on, it became apparent that the majority of participants had complete trust in our ability to protect their anonymity, and to treat their contributions appropriately. Although the Ethics Committee could not take over the responsibility, it provided me with the overall advice and support that was needed regarding the running of the Study. It was a group of experts from a variety of backgrounds to whom I could take my worries and uncertainties, and get considered and wise opinions. Nowadays, it is assumed that ethics committees need to be independent – I am not sure why. If the aim is to ensure that a study is carried out ethically, surely the optimum is to work with the study to derive solutions to ethical dilemmas, rather than being a jury stating 'yes' or 'no'?

The Study has succeeded, in spite of all odds. This is due to the amazing staff who were involved and were particularly important in making sure that the Study ran smoothly and within appropriate ethical limits, as well as the members of the Ethics Committee who had major beneficial impacts on the ways in which the data were collected and used. When persuading Karen to write this book, I asked her to ensure that she considered the triumphs and failures 'warts and all' – she has done so admirably (as anticipated). It was important to document where it could have been improved and where it fulfilled its aims so that others may learn from both. This document tells the story of this pioneering, informative and rewarding enterprise.

*Jean Golding*
*Bristol, August 2017*

# Preface

The Avon Longitudinal Study of Parents and Children (ALSPAC), also known as 'Children of the 90s', is an internationally renowned longitudinal birth cohort study, based within the University of Bristol in South-West England. ALSPAC's main goal, in collaboration with local, national and international scientists, is to understand the ways in which the physical and social environment interact, over time, with genetic inheritance to affect health, behaviour and development. Over 14,000 pregnant women were enrolled during 1991–92 and these mothers, with their partners and children and, more recently, others from their extended families, continue to give vast amounts of data: physical, psychological, social, educational, environmental, biological and genetic. The collection and analysis of these unique, diverse and complex data sets raised many ethical concerns, and from the outset, it became clear that sound ethical and legal advice would be necessary to guarantee appropriate protection for the Study participants, including those yet to be born.

At the time ALSPAC was established, there were no guidelines for the ethical governance of such longitudinal studies and no other ethics committees dealing with these issues, so ALSPAC founded its own pioneering ethics committee – the ALSPAC Ethics and Law Committee. This was the first ethics committee attached to a longitudinal study and the first to deal with the ethical issues arising from the collection of genetic material from a population sample. This aspect of the study design was a research methodology not used before; genetic studies had previously been preoccupied with 'pedigrees' and individual inheritance. ALSPAC was also the first comprehensive birth cohort to enrol participants in utero and to include fathers or partners in the Study from the outset.

The aim of this book is to describe the innovative work carried out by the ALSPAC Committee in its early years, particularly how the core ethical principles were established and then how the policies evolved as the Study progressed and became more complex as the children grew up and as the interest and understanding of the ethics of such studies developed and advanced in academia, politics and beyond. This book should be of interest to all those curious about the development of ethical protection for participants within longitudinal studies, not only ethicists, epidemiologists, historians and other academics, but also professionals and lay members of research ethics committees and any individual who is, or has been, a participant in longitudinal epidemiological research.

The book is enlivened by quotes from Committee members that have been interviewed recently, who reflect not only on the pioneering work of the Committee, but also on the unusual style and inspirational leadership of the first Committee Chair, Professor Michael Furmston. The first part of the book documents this unusual style, the changing status of the Committee as research governance developed within the University and the National Health Service (NHS), and, with it, the sometimes difficult relationship with these other official bodies.

The second part of the book describes policy development, with separate chapters detailing:

- Confidentiality and anonymisation: the complexities of providing a secure system when it was essential to link individual participants' ongoing sequential data. Deductive disclosure was a particular concern in such a localised study.
- Informed consent: the practical considerations of all aspects of consent and assent, including implied, withdrawal, proxy, dual (parent and child), sole (child only) and, most controversial, 'broad' consent for the use of genetic material. Too much information was considered as detrimental as too little.

- Child protection: the principle of non-intervention that was inherent in the design of ALSPAC was soon challenged as child protection concerns arose when Study families were visited at home, attended ALSPAC research clinics or imparted worrying information when interviewed or answering questionnaires. Intervention could also involve breaking the guarantee of anonymity so essential for the carefully nurtured trust of the participants.
- Disclosure of results: the Committee's general position of non-disclosure was also challenged with the detection of treatable conditions either foreseen (such as anaemia) or incidental (such as tumours).
- Disclosure of individuals' results on request: the Committee reviewed all requests on a case-by-case basis but despite conflicting legal opinions and considerable pressure, they never felt an individual's circumstances warranted disclosure and, with it, the risks of breaking the guarantee of anonymity.
- Requests for help by individual participants: requests for help, sometimes quite harrowing, were also reviewed on a case-by-case basis and, very occasionally, the guarantee of anonymity was broken on compassionate grounds.
- Linkage to third-party databases: opt-out consent was initially acceptable but this became inadequate over time as more comprehensive protection of patients became obligatory and complex procedures had to be negotiated.

Although these chapters cover familiar concepts within the now well-established discipline of medical ethics, the ALSPAC Committee was at the forefront of ethical thinking in regard to genetic epidemiology and longitudinal studies. How much the Committee's work contributed to the current debates on these issues, evident in the abundance of journals and publications on the ethics of research, is debatable and references within this book have been limited to the few with obvious relevance. The Committee had to work from first principles and grapple with the real ethical dilemmas that emerged as the Study progressed and became ever more complex. Many of the policies arising from these deliberations are considered standard practice within medical research now, others remain controversial. Nevertheless, these principles and policies have served ALSPAC well, with the integrity of the Study never compromised.

The final part of the book describes the broader remit of the Committee when deliberating on the ethical issues that arose when endeavouring to reduce attrition rates with appropriate incentives or collaborating with commercial companies. The Committee also had unique oversight of the whole of ALSPAC as it reviewed in detail all that was asked of participants. Finally, the wider influence of the Committee is discussed, not only in a formal advisory capacity for other institutions, such as a House of Lords Science and Technology Sub-Committee and the European Society of Human Genetics, but also as an exemplar for other longitudinal studies, a research methodology that has become increasingly popular since ALSPAC began. These interventions and the importance of the Committee's work beyond that of protecting the Study participants have not been documented previously, although some references can be found scattered within the Committee minutes. The extensive influence of the Committee should provide weight to those considering the Committee's work in the light of their own.

## Personal perspective

In describing the early days of the Committee, a completely objective perspective was not possible as I have not been a detached observer. As a recent and thoroughly sleep-deprived mother, I joined Jean Golding's Unit of Paediatric and Perinatal Epidemiology in 1988 as a medical coder when ALSPAC was being planned. As with all staff within ALSPAC in the early days, I had a variety of simultaneous roles, mainly related to my nursing background. In 1998, Jean asked me to complete the local NHS Research Ethics Committee form for approval for the first all-cohort research clinic, and so began my involvement with the ethical issues within ALSPAC. A year later, I was asked to take the minutes for the Committee, and soon after that, I became the Committee Secretary and then the ALSPAC Ethics Manager. For over 14 years I worked closely with the Committee, some members have become friends and I continue to work with Jean Golding. Other than verbatim quotes from recorded interviews and extracts from the Committee minutes, opinions and any errors remain my own.

There have been three main sources used when writing this document:

1. Minutes and accompanying documents of the Committee between its establishment in 1990 and July 2005, when the retirement of Jean Golding was formally acknowledged by the Committee. Ethical approval was given for the deposit of this material as a public resource in the University of Bristol ALSPAC Administrative Archive held by the Library's Special Collections (Committee reference E201301, July 2015).
2. Papers during the same period from: Jean Golding; Michael Furmston, Chair of the Committee throughout this period; Elizabeth Mumford (née Roberts), Secretary of the Committee for the first 10 years; and myself, Secretary of the Committee for the following 14 years.
3. Brief oral histories recorded by me during 2012–13 from eight members of the Committee, as well as Professor Marcus Pembrey, ALSPAC's Director of Genetics, who was central to the inclusion of genetics from the outset in ALSPAC's design and provided essential information and advice to the Committee.

These documents have been indexed and will be archived along with the videotaped oral histories in the University of Bristol Special Collections as the ALSPAC Ethics Archive, a subset of the main ALSPAC Administrative Archive that provides a rich resource for further research into the origins and complex methodology of this extraordinarily ambitious and successful study.

*Karen Birmingham*
*August 2017*

# Introduction

The Avon Longitudinal Study of Parents and Children (ALSPAC) was part of a European consortium of longitudinal birth cohorts, designed by Jean Golding, who had extensive knowledge and experience of such studies from working on the previous UK national birth cohorts. It was an immensely ambitious study that uniquely included genetics in its methodology and was supported by a Steering Committee who believed, unlike many people, that Jean's vision could be achieved. They also believed that it was vital for the Study to be beyond criticism not only scientifically, but also ethically, and promoted the novel concept of an ethics committee attached to the Study itself – the ALSPAC Ethics and Law Committee. To insist on such thorough and ongoing ethical review was exceptional at a time when research governance was minimal and ethical scrutiny not obligatory. ALSPAC's frequent and detailed data collections from diverse sources (self-completion questionnaires, interviews, hands-on measurements, biological samples and environmental measures) provided a unique and complex resource for scientists of many disciplines but also created numerous ethical issues not encountered previously. It would be the Committee's task to identify the principles and design the policies that would provide comprehensive protection of the Cohort throughout the Study.

The Avon Longitudinal Study of Parents and Children is known to the scientific community as ALSPAC and to the Study participants and public as 'Children of the 90s'.[1] ALSPAC was based in the UK city of Bristol and the surrounding area but was part of a multi-centre European consortium (the European Study of Pregnancy and Childhood [ELSPAC]) (Golding, 1989a), which was initiated after a meeting in Moscow in 1985 convened by the World Health

Organisation. Jean Golding was the initial Director of both ELSPAC and ALSPAC and brought with her a resolute belief in the value of longitudinal birth cohorts, based substantially on her previous work on the 1958 and 1970 UK national birth cohorts.[2]

The aims of ALSPAC were exceptionally ambitious: to identify the ways in which to optimise the health and development of children.[3] Not only were detailed and frequent data collections planned, but several innovative components were also included: to collect genetic data from the outset; to recruit women in pregnancy; and to collect data from both the mothers and their partners. George Davey Smith, Professor of Clinical Epidemiology, who took over from Jean Golding as Scientific Director of ALSPAC when she retired, has frequently talked about his first reaction to ALSPAC. In August 1989, he noticed a brief paragraph by Jean Golding in the back of the *Lancet* (Golding, 1989b) describing ALSPAC and asking for potential collaborators to make contact. He considered the project an impossible undertaking, dismissed it out of hand and, not yet knowing Jean Golding personally, thought it sounded implausibly ambitious. If studying children was not ambitious enough, ALSPAC rapidly expanded to include adults and, to reflect this, in 1999, the meaning of the acronym ALSPAC was adapted from 'Pregnancy and Childhood' to the current 'Parents and Children'.

From her experience with other longitudinal studies, Jean Golding knew of the difficulties of analysing and interpreting large longitudinal data sets that lack sufficient detail to obtain robust results. This, combined with a chance meeting in Athens in 1988 with Professor Marcus Pembrey (Overy et al, 2012, p 11), Professor of Paediatric Genetics at the Institute of Child Health in London, resulted in ALSPAC being designed to incorporate genetic data as well as the detailed and frequent physical, psychological, social, educational, environmental and biological measures originally planned. Marcus Pembrey reflected on the significance and context of this methodology when interviewed in 2013:

"It was fairly clear that by 1988, it [the Human Genome Project[4]] was going to happen.… So, I knew that the big challenge – which no one really knew what the hell was going on – was these common diseases, the genetic component of asthma, allergy, diabetes, you name it.… It seemed a good plan." (Marcus Pembrey, Oral History Interview, 2013)

A good plan indeed, also described as an "audacious plan"[5] by the late Professor David Baum, the charismatic Head of the Department of Child Health at the University of Bristol at the time and a stalwart supporter of ALSPAC from the very beginning. David Baum was "a man who had a hundred ideas a day", as described by his friend and colleague Dr Timothy Chambers, also interviewed in 2013, who went on to say:

"I don't think David Baum had had a major focus on epidemiology … I think David came under the influence of Jean [Golding], quite rightly. David being David, once he was seized with something would then take the very big view … Jean had had the idea, it wouldn't have taken much for David to be galvanised by it and to use his influence alongside hers to promote it.… Who could not be fired up with enthusiasm for David's breathtaking visions?" (Tim Chambers, Oral History Interview, 2013)

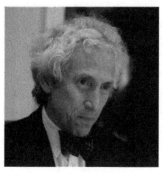

David Baum

The description of ALSPAC as audacious was baffling to Dr David Jewell, ALSPAC Ethics and Law Committee Chair from 2010 to 2013 but a member of the Committee for 10 years previously, who admitted when interviewed that it took over a decade to understand why the Study could be considered audacious:

> "I didn't quite understand why [audacious], but it [ALSPAC] now seems both farsighted as well as everything else…. The genetics looked just about possible but a long way into the future and it now is becoming apparent that it has happened a lot quicker than anyone ever expected, so other studies now are trying to emulate what ALSPAC had built into its own 'genes' at the very beginning." (David Jewell, Oral History Interview, 2012)

The Study planned to enrol as many pregnant women as possible over a period of one year within the defined catchment area of three Avon Health Districts.[6] Follow-up of these mothers, their Study children and their partners with detailed data collections was anticipated for at least seven years. As the Study progressed, so the design expanded. Over 14,000 mothers were recruited during 1990–92, a longer enrolment period than first anticipated, with data collected from five main sources: self-completion postal questionnaires; hands-on measurements; biological samples; third-party sources, such as hospital and educational records; and environmental monitoring, such as air quality. The longitudinal aspect of the Study became inestimable; seven years became lifelong and 650 of the children's children have (as of August 2017) been recruited to a third-generational study. The mothers received four questionnaires during pregnancy and by the time Jean Golding retired, 80 different questionnaires had been sent to Study participants. These questionnaires could be up to 60 pages long. The hands-on measurements began with 'Children in Focus', involving approximately 1,400 children who attended research clinics, initially at the age of four months and then nine more times in their first five years. This expanded to annual half-day clinics for all Cohort children from the age of seven to 13 years, with over 8,000 children seen at seven years and just over 6,000 at 13 years. Annual clinics overlapped as the Cohort comprised mothers whose births were due over a 21-month period. The collection of biological samples included placentas, blood, saliva, urine, hair, nails and teeth; DNA was extracted and cell lines eventually created, enabling infinite supplies of DNA. This has become a unique, internationally recognised resource used by thousands of collaborators from a multitude of disciplines.

There were no ethical committees in the UK specifically concerned with longitudinal studies at the time, despite the UK pioneering national birth cohorts in 1946, 1958 and 1970. So, in 1989, while ALSPAC was still being planned and piloted, the ALSPAC Steering Committee, which included David Baum, initiated an ethics advisory committee attached to the Study itself. As Elizabeth Mumford, lawyer and first Secretary of the ALSPAC Committee said:

> "… it is ground-breaking that the founders of ALSPAC had this idea, not of submitting reluctantly to scrutiny, but actually asking for help and collaboration. That is the really outstanding thing about the beginning of this Committee: the sense that having an ethically ideal study was every bit as important as having a scientifically ideal study." (History of ALSPAC c 1980–2000, Wellcome Witnesses to 20th Century Medicine, 2012, p 72)

This Committee had to grapple with the unfamiliar issues arising from not only an exceptionally long study (lifetimes in fact), but also enrolling participants in utero and the collection and utilisation of genetic data. Genetic issues had hardly been addressed previously in the context of population studies, in contrast to clinical genetics. There was little guidance: no other ethical committees within the University of Bristol (the University Ethics of Research Committee was only established in 2002), no academic department for ethics (the University Centre for Ethics in Medicine was established in 1998) and limited degrees of expertise or interest in the local National Health Service (NHS) Research Ethics Committees (LRECs). These committees, based in each NHS Area Health Authority, were formally delegated the responsibility for ethical review of NHS research by the Department of Health, although guidelines making these NHS committees obligatory were not published until the year after the ALSPAC Committee was set up.[7]

The early years were taken up with formulating principles and establishing processes to ensure comprehensive protection of the ALSPAC participants. Consideration of the implications of enrolling participants from a local community was paramount. Not only would many of the participants know each other, but they might know some of the staff too. Quite a few ALSPAC staff were also participants, which complicated matters further. The guarantee of anonymity was essential to the Committee; a guarantee of mere confidentiality would not be adequate. Establishing participants' trust in this respect was considered essential if attrition rates were to be kept low and data from questionnaires were to be credible. Yet, absolute and irreversible anonymity is not possible in a longitudinal study, not least because individuals' data collected at sequential time points have to be linked. The Study participants were told 'we shall be using two separate computers in this study, one to store personal identifiers and the other for survey results'.[8] Computers were in their infancy; Jean Golding's pre-computer 'punchcards' from her earlier epidemiological work were still to be found in her office and not just for historical interest. Innovative computing and administrative structures, now considered cumbersome, had to be designed by the ALSPAC Computing Manager to safeguard this guarantee as far as possible. This did not prevent the Committee having to reconsider this assurance time and time and time again when confronted by the real issues arising as the Study progressed, such as feedback to individuals of their test results or the protection of vulnerable children.

The Committee took into consideration not only the protection of Study participants, but also the protection of staff and of ALSPAC's and the University's reputation. The Committee rapidly became vital to the governance of ALSPAC as, in the early years, neither the University nor the LRECs had formalised their own governance procedures. As

Richard Ashcroft, Professor of Bioethics and one-time member of the Committee, said:

> "... the Committee in my time were very clear about the need for ALSPAC not only to be ethically sound, but also to be *seen* to be ethically sound, and it took its advisory responsibilities very seriously. [Although] not involved in the day-to-day management ... they are responsible if anything goes wrong.... When called upon to give advice about policy matters, it gave solid advice as far as I know and certainly hasn't had any major [ethical] problems." (Richard Ashcroft, Oral History Interview, 2013)

To be ethically sound with no major calamities was quite a feat for such an audacious study. How much this was due to the solid advice of the ALSPAC Ethics and Law Committee is disputable, even among the Committee members themselves. However, Jean Golding remains convinced that the Committee was crucial to the overall success of the Study.

# Part One
# ALSPAC Ethics and Law Committee:
## a new concept

# ONE

# Preliminaries and pioneers: framing the questions

The inspirational concept of an ethics and law committee attached to ALSPAC was initiated by a few key individuals at a time when there was a scarcity of guidelines and minimal formal governance and when research ethics committees were in their infancy. The appointment of lawyers as both Chair and Secretary to the Committee was crucial in providing sound legal advice for the pioneering work that was conducted without any framework for ethical practice in this type of genetic epidemiological research. Although the principle of anonymity was paramount, identifying the issues and formulating the questions to establish broader principles was necessary before policies could be established.

The ALSPAC Ethics and Law Committee was initiated in 1989 by the late Professor David Baum, founding member of the ALSPAC Steering Committee and, at the time, head of his newly established Institute of Child Health at the University of Bristol. The small ALSPAC Steering Committee (see Appendix 1) welcomed David Baum's novel suggestion of an ethics committee attached to the Study itself. Included on the Steering Committee were two members of the Institute of Child Health in London: Catherine Peckham, Professor of Paediatric Epidemiology, who had a particular interest in, and experience of, working with birth cohort studies; and Marcus Pembrey, Professor of

Paediatric Genetics, whose vision for ALSPAC as a longitudinal *genetic* study cannot be underestimated. A population study that included studying the environmental and genetic interactions related to common diseases was entirely original.

All on the Steering Committee recognised that the genetic aspects of the Study in particular would have ethical implications that had not been considered in this context before. In the briefest of memos, 'Ethical considerations for the ALSPAC' (see Figure 1), David Baum suggested that ALSPAC should have its own committee to 'serve as guardians of the ethical principles'. Two principles were outlined:

> Maintaining the absolute confidentiality of the data base and establishing the principle of non-attributability of the data to named families both now and in the future.

> Similarly, establishing the absolute principle of non-attributability of the data relating to the mother and baby cell lines. (David Baum, memo, November 1989)

Although the inclusion of cell lines (used for the production of unlimited DNA) was an inspired and integral part of ALSPAC's design, albeit raising significant ethical issues, it took until 1996 for Jean Golding and Marcus Pembrey to persuade any funders to support this aspect of the Study.

## Figure 1: David Baum's memo, November 1989

23 NOV. HIL

DRAFT

### ETHICAL CONSIDERATIONS FOR THE ALSPAC

Securing the support of the three district Ethical Committees for the study in principle and the detailed projects.

Maintaining the absolute confidentiality of the data base and establishing the principle of non-attributabilty of the data to named families both now and in the future.

Similarly, establishing the absolute principle of non-attributability of the data relating to the mother and baby cell lines.

The appointment of a committee to represent the community's views on the project as a whole, but most notably to serve as guardians of the ethical principles. Such committee to include representatives of certain groups: parents, community health councils, health, education and social services, and University representatives from the faculties of Law, Philosophy, Theology. Possibly inviting Professor Furmston to act as committee Chairman.

Charging the committee with the task of producing a pro-active document and public statement addressing in full, ethical aspects of the study and the safe-guarding of the public's interest in the broadest possible terms.

JDB.
24.11.89.

So, the Ethics and Law Committee was established in April 1990, with Michael Furmston, Professor of Law at the University, as Chair, another lawyer, Elizabeth Mumford (née Roberts), a specialist in medical law, as Secretary, plus a variety of experts from other disciplines (see Box 1) who were selected by Michael Furmston in consultation with David Baum. As Gordon Stirrat, Professor of Obstetrics and Gynaecology, a founding member of both the Steering and Ethics Committees, recalled "getting Michael involved was a stroke of genius because of his status and because of the fact he brought *the law* into it, which is so important. It was an ethics *and law* committee, wasn't just an ethics committee".[1]

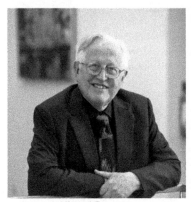

Michael Furmston

It was another stroke of genius, but this time on Michael Furmston's part, to get Elizabeth Mumford involved. As she explained, referring to herself:

> "Michael was a brilliant lawyer and had an enormous range of knowledge but I think he thought it might be important to have somebody who had a particular interest and expertise in medical law and medical ethics. It was quite a new area of the law, which was rapidly developing at that point and still is, and I think he thought it interesting to have somebody who was probably fairly junior and who would go off and look up

the things that were necessary and fill in the details." (Elizabeth Mumford, Oral History Interview, 2013)

Elizabeth Mumford, with her "good legal mind", had done the Committee's "groundwork" thoroughly, as related by Richard Ashcroft, the ethicist on the Committee at the time, who went on to describe the Committee's approach to ethical issues:

"[The Committee was] not quite what I was used to in that it was legally driven, with both Michael Furmston and Elizabeth Mumford on the Committee ... from the very beginning, with Alastair [Campbell, Professor of Medical Ethics] and myself only joining later ... but it was quite different from a National Health Service ethics committee in that those committees tend to be very medically orientated and also were, and still are, advised *not* to think of themselves as giving legal advice. So, there were some quite important cultural differences." (Richard Ashcroft, Oral History Interview, 2013)

As Richard Ashcroft inferred, there were cultural distinctions other than being legally driven, such as Study participants being included on the Committee and the Chair's unique style. Although Michael Furmston's expertise was in contract law, he was considered not only "wise",[2] but also a "wise choice",[3] generating much admiration and affection from many of the other Committee members. As Elizabeth Mumford described:

"... he is a man who is 'larger than life' in every way. He was twice dean of the Bristol law faculty, he was Pro Vice Chancellor, and eminent scholar in contract and commercial law, areas of law miles away from this one. He was a barrister, a practising barrister. He would lead the meetings in a style, which I suppose is reminiscent of the development of the common law, so he would do it by stories and anecdotes. Some of them were anecdotes about his own home life – quite a lot of them were – but his home life was rather interesting as well. He had 10 children plus about 22 dogs, and goats.... He was a postal chess champion. He was an expert on the American Civil War and on cricket.... But he was enthusiastic, he was warm, he was encouraging and he had a wonderful style of leading meetings. So, it made a very civilised, very enjoyable atmosphere in which to conduct some really very difficult business."(History of ALSPAC c. 1980–2000, Wellcome Witnesses to 20th Century Medicine, 2012, p 74)

## Box 1: ALSPAC Ethics and Law Committee: founding members

Professor Michael Furmston, Chair, Department of Law, University of Bristol

Professor David Baum, Institute of Child Health, University of Bristol

Professor Gordon Stirrat, Department of Obstetrics & Gynaecology, University of Bristol

Professor Peter Keen, Dean, Faculty of Medicine, University of Bristol

Professor Ursula King, Department of Theology, University of Bristol

Dr Iain Lister Cheese, Senior Medical Officer, Department of Health, London

Dr Timothy Chambers, Consultant Paediatrician, Southmead Hospital, Bristol

Mr David Hirschmann, Department of Philosophy, University of Bristol

Miss Elizabeth Roberts, Secretary, Department of Law, University of Bristol (to become Mrs Elizabeth Mumford in 1995)

Dr Jean Golding, Institute of Child Health, University of Bristol

David Baum, Jean Golding and Gordon Stirrat were members of both the ALSPAC Steering Committee and the Ethics and Law Committee, and therefore provided a direct conduit between these Committees in the early years of ALSPAC when the complex practicalities of setting up the Study were being planned and implemented. As envisioned by David Baum, the Ethics and Law Committee was multidisciplinary. The range of expertise within the Committee allowed for a sound scientific grasp of most proposals by at least some members, who could then explain to the others if necessary. Jean Golding was always a vital source of information and scientific explanation too. In general, scientific review of projects was for the Scientific Advisory Committee, which had overall control of the projects that were undertaken. For this, they took advice from experts in the field, including other ALSPAC advisory committees, such as the Genetic Advisory Committee, thus securing the scientific integrity of the projects carried out. Although the Ethics and Law Committee tried *not* to review the science of proposals, they were inevitably concerned with their value as they had to balance this with the impact on participants in terms of time, inconvenience and risk. As David Jewell reflected when considering whether ethics committees should concern themselves with scientific review:

"… are the participants being asked to give up their time to answer a question that either has been answered already, or isn't worth asking, or isn't going to come to an answer because you are not going to get enough of them to participate? All of those are things [that] would be perfectly legitimate areas of concern for an ethics committee." (David Jewell, Oral History Interview, 2012)

The input of Study participants to the Committee's deliberations was of great importance. David Baum had suggested that participants should be on the Committee in 1989, but it was not until December 1994, when the Study children were between two and three years old, that the first Study mother (Mrs Sheila Bryer) joined the Committee. The inclusion of Study mothers as "representative parents, able to reflect things that would actually bother other parents",[4] was incomprehensible to some other researchers who "even today [think] why on earth you could possibly want a lay person on the Committee?".[5] Yet, as another member of the Committee described, "This came through again and again, this was a *shared* enterprise: professionals, clinical professionals, health professional and lay people".[6]

As Elizabeth Mumford (1999a) describes in her first paper on the Committee's early work, there was little in English law relating to medical research and the guidance in international codes or from professional bodies was of little relevance to studies such as ALSPAC. Priorities when protecting human research subjects as stipulated by the Declaration of Helsinki (World Medical Association, 1964) are subtly different in epidemiology from those in clinical medicine. The guidelines of the Council for International Organizations of Medical Sciences (CIOMS, 1991), which did provide an ethical framework specifically for epidemiological research, were not published until after the Committee had been established. Therefore, the ALSPAC Committee's pioneering work was conducted without a framework for ethical practice in this type of scientific research. The fundamental ethical policies were formulated mainly in the first few meetings of the Committee's existence but evolved over many years as ethical issues arose and were brought before the Committee. This process was described by both Michael Furmston and Elizabeth Mumford as similar to the English legal system:

"The development of the rules was what I would regard as characteristic of English case law development, which [when] we had a particular problem, we kicked it around and came up with what we thought was the right solution.... And then if we got a similar problem, we would look back and see what we did last time and consider it in the light of that." (Michael Furmston, Oral History Interview, 2012)

"It was like our 'constitution', it's not written but everyone knew ... because there was a fairly high degree of consistency in the early days of Committee meetings, so we all knew we'd sat there, we'd gone through it, we'd come up with these conclusions and that's what we referred to and when we started later on getting individual issues, so we said, 'Well this is how we had discussed it, does it apply?'.... So, we couldn't do this, wouldn't do that, let's refer to what we said, we'd go back to the minutes, go back to our own discussions, our own memories of our own discussions. So, it was like a constitution ... We had this sort of loose structure, if you want to call it a 'constitution', and then we developed things incrementally so we didn't look at ... hypothetical cases, we looked at real cases and then we would build on those in the same way that the common law develops." (Elizabeth Mumford, Oral History Interview, 2012)

Working without any relevant guidelines or formal governance structures in those early days, the Committee was not always consistent. Relying on the Committee members' memories of 'the rules' rather than documenting policies was not foolproof, especially as the years rolled by and the Study became increasingly complex. It is difficult to discern if the lack of documentation was due to the ambiguous status of the Committee, which evolved from advisory to something more formal, or to the ad hoc nature of the Committee, which catalysed Tim Chambers's resignation, as described in Chapter Two. Yet, some policies did appear in the minutes, such as the ones to protect the confidentiality of participants selected for sub-studies known as 'the 500 rule'[7] (Mumford, 1999b). This rule was put in place to safeguard the anonymity of participants who were to be studied as part of subgroups selected on the basis of answers to questionnaires. It was decided that any subgroup identified for further study would have to be matched by at least an equal number of controls and that the total number would have to be at least 500. Other policies appeared in a variety of forms, including guidelines for specific groups of staff, such as interviewers visiting participants' homes to help complete questionnaires,[8] or rules for data handling and processing.[9] These seemingly haphazard arrangements were more robust than might be imagined and seemed to work well. The ethical principles, especially David Baum's first principle of 'non-attributability of the data to named families' and the mechanism involved (known as the Ethical Divide, described in detail in Chapter Five) were part of the culture of all ALSPAC staff. As with the Ethics Committee, the low turnover (and initially relatively small number) of ALSPAC staff, who were renowned for their loyalty to Jean Golding and the Study, enabled the ethical principles and policies to be understood without formal documentation. This relaxed attitude to the crucial ethical underpinning of the Study would not be acceptable today and towards the end of Michael Furmston's Chairmanship, policies began to be formally documented. At much the same time, the University also began to formalise their policies concerning the ethics of research.

Jean Golding, as Director of ALSPAC, attended, almost without exception, all the Committee meetings (up to 13 per year) in the first 16 years (as did Michael Furmston) in order to provide information and listen to the Committee's deliberations. When questioned about her role on the Committee by funding bodies and others, she was sometimes classified as an 'observer' or Michael Furmston was known to have said that she was not considered a 'voting member'. This was hardly relevant as voting was never considered an appropriate way to make decisions during Michael Furmston's 16 years as Chair. Her position on the Committee was crucial. It was taken on trust that she would bring to the Committee any relevant issues arising during the running of the Study, allowing the Committee to formulate consistent policies, even if not formally documented, on which the Study would continue. The Committee also took it on trust that not only she, but also the ALSPAC staff and collaborators, would act on the Committee's advice. This did not always happen, as will be seen, but usually only due to error rather than conscious rebellion.

Most members of the Committee served for many years (see Appendix 2); some left when other work became onerous but returned to the Committee at a later date. The lengthy terms served were vital to the culture and modus operandi. It enabled members to have a comprehensive grasp not only of what was asked of the participants, but also of the reasoning involved in constructing the 'constitution'. It also contributed to the relaxed cohesion that developed within the Committee, allowing members' discussions to be "formal but not hierarchical",[10] with conflicting views expressed without inhibitions. This longevity of service is frequently considered unacceptable now, with many bodies stipulating a limited term for membership or holding official committee positions such as chair or secretary, although the reasoning behind this remains obscure.

There was no formal training in ethics for Committee members in the first 16 years, which certainly surprised members of the Committee who joined later,[11] although David Jewell explained that "It is not surprising in a way that other people weren't able to say at the beginning 'this is what we expect of you' [as] it was only very slowly that I began to understand how the Committee worked".[12] David Baum had tried to seek advice as early as May 1990, 'particularly looking for problem areas which we may not as yet have addressed',[13] when he approached Colin Normand, Chair of the British Paediatric Association Ethics Advisory Committee. Although Professor Normand indicated that his Committee 'would be very interested to consider in a general way the implications of … longitudinal studies of this sort', there is no evidence that this was taken any further.[14] The University of Bristol Centre for Ethics in Medicine now provides training for NHS and University research ethics committees, as well as for other academic, health-care and legal professionals, using ALSPAC as an exemplar.[15] The Centre was one of the first providers of such training courses in the UK but it was not established until 1998, many years after the ALSPAC Committee had been founded. This indicates the extent to which the Committee was exploring unfamiliar territory, having to formulate the appropriate questions to be asked and principles on which the Study should be run.

Terms of reference for the Committee were produced by Michael Furmston when pressed by Jean Golding's successors at the very end of his term as Chair. In contrast to the current 14-page document, he produced four brief items:

1. To consider the general principles which should govern the conduct of the study, in particular to formulate guidelines on the key questions of consent and confidentiality;
2. To keep this process under constant review;
3. To consider ethical and legal problems arising from the conduct of the study;
4. To consider other questions on which its advice is sought. (ALSPAC Ethics and Law Committee, 'Terms of reference', 2006)

Despite this apparent administrative oversight, it seemed clear that protection of the participants in the broadest sense was the Committee's paramount concern and, as David Baum had stated, 'to serve as guardians of the ethical principles'. Perhaps not obvious to David Baum at the time, the Committee first had to identify the issues, formulate the pertinent questions and then establish the ethical principles.

# TWO

# Informal or casual: an unusual style

Michael Furmston's unusual style of conducting the meetings, with his warm informality and many entertaining and highly relevant anecdotes, did not detract from the Committee's recognition of the importance of the work to be done. This generated a remarkable commitment in the Committee members, evident in the longevity of membership. With no terms of reference, defined status or formal documentation of policies (other than in the narrative minutes that detailed the essence of the discussions), the Committee today would not be considered acceptable, yet the calibre and conscientiousness of the members, with their considered contributions, produced effective governance and robust protection of the Study participants throughout.

The style of the ALSPAC Ethics and Law Committee under Michael Furmston's leadership was particularly unusual, as recounted by those Committee members who had, in their professional capacities, considerable experience of university, National Health Service (NHS) or other committees. Michael Furmston himself remembers the meetings as being "not elaborately structured", but with "serious, well-informed discussions" that were "interesting and intellectually demanding".[1] This was echoed by two founding members of the Committee, Tim Chambers, Consultant Paediatrician, who described the meetings as "immensely stimulating",[2] and Ian Lister Cheese,

Senior Medical Officer in the Department of Health, who pointed out "… the keenness, enthusiasm, the sense of duty and responsibility that all the members brought. There was that sense of something important to be done".[3] Richard Ashcroft remembered that "some of the discussions could be quite heated because difficult decisions were being made but it was always collegial".[4] The Committee's modus operandi was set by Michael Furmston, who, as Jean Golding described, was "such a very warm, friendly, exciting and different personality that the whole Committee took on the role of being friendly and exciting and positive in its thinking".[5] Yet, his Chairmanship was:

"… deceptive, you could look at it and think 'What on earth?', it is all very informal and he's not a very good Chairman, but actually, when you got into it, you saw his style was very authoritative, not authoritarian by any means, but he was absorbing everything, then, not the killer question, the critical question would come out." (Tim Chambers, Oral History Interview, 2013)

David Jewell elaborated on this disarming technique:

"When Michael could see some glaring fallacy in what somebody [a visiting researcher or collaborator, not one of the Committee] was saying, he always used to say 'Do you mind if I ask an idiot-boy question?'. And we [the Committee] learned by this stage that when he said this, he was going to say something completely devastating." (David Jewell, Oral History Interview, 2012)

Michael Furmston's anecdotal style was legendary too. As Elizabeth Mumford described:

"… *he* was like the common law, he was very anecdotal, he would say 'Well this reminds me of such and such' and if you were a busy person thinking 'Oh please, get to the point', you might find this rather frustrating, but, actually, he would hone it down to the point. This story was there for a purpose.... He did it well but because it was this slightly roundabout way of coming at business, it could discourage some people, but I think it contributed to the friendliness of the Committee, and the fact we all felt comfortable with one another meant that we made better decisions." (Elizabeth Mumford, Oral History Interview, 2013)

The "respectable sandwich lunch"[6] may seem unimportant but it was thought that it contributed not only to people feeling comfortable, but also to people attending the meetings relatively consistently. Jean Golding recalled that "It was a committee people wanted to attend so it's one of the few committees I've ever been on where the attendance was very high. We didn't pay anybody. We provided a good lunch but that was it".[7]

Richard Ashcroft, contrary to most others who emphasised the Committee's informality, found his first few meetings:

"... quite intimidating actually, not in the sense that I wasn't made welcome, because I was, but it was a quite formal committee, the personalities were quite formal, Jean is quite formal and Michael Furmston is quite formal, very lawyerly in an old-school way, quite charming when you get to know him but off-putting if you are not used to that sort of person and I wasn't." (Richard Ashcroft, Oral History Interview, 2013)

The Committee's role as an advisory committee supporting Jean Golding was acknowledged by many, not least by Jean herself, although Elizabeth Mumford expressed some reservations:

"The feeling was we were friends sitting around the table. Jean was there. She was the Head of the Study, she wasn't a member of the Committee, but she was there at all the meetings and the feeling was that we were helping her, that we were all working together, maybe too much at times, maybe there was too much of a link and we felt that we were talking about *us* in the sense not as an ethics committee, but *us* in the sense of the Study. Maybe we should have been slightly more removed from it but I don't think that blurred our judgement in any way." (Elizabeth Mumford, Oral History Interview, 2013)

Perhaps what was not acknowledged or even noticed at that time was that although the male to female ratio in the Committee gradually became fairly even after the initial ratio of 7:3, the Committee was made up entirely of white, middle-class professionals. The feeling of 'friends sitting around a table' might be due, in part, to the Committee comprising a broadly homogeneous group. David Baum's vision of the Committee's make-up was extensive but with no suggestion that it should be representative of the Cohort as such. He had suggested: 'The appointment of a committee to represent the community's views on the project as a whole…. Such committee to include representatives of certain groups: parents, community health councils, health, education and social services, and University representatives from the faculties of Law, Philosophy and Theology.'[8]

It took many years for these various groups to be represented on the Committee, and community health councils and social services never were. Minority ethnic groups were also not represented, but Bristol and the surrounding areas did not have large populations of minority ethnic groups. The 1991 UK Census reported that 4.1% of mothers with infants less than a year old described themselves as non-white (compared with 7.6% of mothers across the whole of the UK), with only 2.2% ALSPAC mothers described as such (Fraser et al, 2012).

## Study participants

Despite David Baum's far-sighted suggestion to include parents on the Committee when he initially outlined the composition of the Committee, Study mothers were only invited on to the Committee after four years and fathers not until 15 years after that, when they were enrolled in their own right. Prior to this, data had been collected from partners only if mothers elected to pass on questionnaires to them. The mothers were selected at the suggestion of other Committee members who knew them and "thought this person would be good".[9] Their importance and value was acknowledged by other Committee members and it seemed they integrated with few problems: "I remember how warmly they were welcomed and how comfortable it seemed to me they felt.... They were listened to and they didn't generate resistance, we were of one mind".[10] Unfortunately, none were available for interview when Committee members were having their brief oral histories recorded, so the Study mothers' recollections are not included here. Richard Ashcroft put into context their role as compared with NHS Research Ethics Committees, who also had lay members:

"So, in a typical ethics committee, you have lay members who are defined by being non-medical and non-university ... whereas the parent members of the ALSPAC Committee had the direct experience of being involved ... in *this* project.... So, in a way, they were more like representatives of the parent body and later of the children as well, where lay members on NHS Research Ethics Committees are *not* representative and they don't have a specific relationship to any particular project.... In fact, if they did, it would be considered that they had a conflict of interests. So, there is an important difference actually. It was something I wondered about from time to time, whether the parent members ... would be more interested in appearing knowledgeable and sensible to *us* than they would be in being good representative parents able to reflect the things that actually would bother other parents. I never saw a case where I thought 'hang on a minute, you've crossed a line here, you are now one of us and that is not what we need you to be'." (Richard Ashcroft, Oral History Interview, 2013)

## Length of service

The longevity of Committee members' service and membership by invitation crucially contributed to the culture and functioning of the Committee, as Gordon Stirrat explained:

"The other quirky aspect of the Committee, which I don't think would be allowed now … is the membership just persisted and persisted and persisted.… It wouldn't be allowed today but, you see, when you had these people with their expertise and they became familiar with the Committee, it worked so well and the alternative of doing the bureaucratic thing of 'Oh, we've got to change them every so often', then some of that folk memory would be lost.… What we did … if we knew there was a need for someone else to come on to the Committee, we thought about it and approached people, we had some discussions and we invited people to come on. I don't think we would be allowed to do that nowadays and, in some ways, that's a shame because it worked well but, you see, no one trusts anyone to self-regulate nowadays." (Gordon Stirrat, Oral History Interview, 2013)

Under Michael Furmston's leadership, the endurance of membership, the friendliness and the lack of hierarchy enabled the Committee to create what one Committee member termed a 'social ecosystem', emphasising the power of such a system 'as the whole [was] greater than the sum of its parts'. He went on to say 'It was the relationship between longstanding members as individuals, beyond just their professional roles, which was so important … the relationship of the Committee to the institution(s) of which it was a part, especially being a vanguard in driving developments and the battles fought.'[11]

Despite, or because of, the anomalies of the Committee set-up, the Committee was judged to have worked well, albeit when judged by members of the Committee itself.

## Minutes

The Committee meeting minutes were also of an unusual style. Elizabeth Mumford, the first Committee Secretary and minute taker, had had experience taking minutes at "… an international committee and because there had been a room full of possibly almost 100 delegates, all making points and all wanting their points to look good, I was fairly used to, not changing things, but certainly working things so they appeared in their best and clearest light on paper."[12] So, her minutes were, in her own words, "creative", she would "fill in the gaps", especially in relation to the law, and try to capture the sense of the discussion that would cover wide-ranging ethical issues. When the author took over as Secretary of the Committee, she took on this style of minutes. She soon discovered that the 'irrelevant' anecdotes, usually Michael Furmston's, after meandering at length, would come right back to the point, as described previously, and so decided to take verbatim notes, which then took much time and effort to write up succinctly and coherently. As the Study became more and more complex, the author often referred to the previous minutes in her role as ALSPAC Ethics Manager. It was useful to be able to inform staff, collaborators or even Committee members how and why the Committee had come to their decisions and the development of their 'policies' going right back to the beginning of the Study.

One Committee member spoke favourably of 'the sense and narrative thread you [the author] bring to the minutes'[13] when referring to the unusual style of minute taking, but they had not always been quite so appreciated. Tim Chambers cited the minutes, which tended not to be circulated in advance and were not formatted in the style usual for current research ethics committees, as one reason for his resignation after seven years on the Committee. His resignation letter to Jean Golding stated:

> By this letter I am also tendering my resignation from the committee. My main reason is that the dates and venues of the meetings make it impossible for me to attend regularly.

I have a subsidiary reason for resigning. The issues discussed by the committee are of the utmost importance and committee members have an accountability for the decisions of the group. I find that the ad hoc arrangements for the committee meetings, the variable punctuality and the haphazard minute taking are below the standards I have met in other ethics committees and I just wonder if they would bear scrutiny if they were held to account.

I apologise for writing in such a forthright way. It would probably have been better to speak to you in person and I will try to do so. Although I have headed this letter 'Private & Confidential' I have done so in order that you would see it first. I would be happy that its contents were divulged to other members of the committee if you thought it right.

I would like to wish ALSPAC the best for the future. It is an exciting and imaginative project. (Tim Chambers, letter to Jean Golding, June 1997)

When reflecting on this so many years later, Tim Chambers did not retract anything that he had written, but clarified that it was not the content of the minutes that concerned him, but that they were circulated on the day of the meeting, with a "sense that it was all rather cobbled together".[14] Elizabeth Mumford was quite open about how she usually wrote them on the day of the meeting but "hope[d] they were not misleading in any way. I put a lot of effort into them even if they were done at the last minute. It was high-intensity last-minute work".[15] Jean Golding expressed similar frustrations to Tim Chambers, "very often, I hadn't taken appropriate notes during the meeting and needed [a] reminder as to what I should be doing, which wasn't always there".[16] When the author became Committee Secretary, she frequently also only just managed to produce the minutes in time for the next meeting but would type up the 'actions' immediately after the meeting and thereby avoided Jean Golding's exasperation.

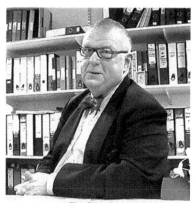
Tim Chambers

Despite Tim Chambers's criticisms when he resigned, he expressed the feelings of many Committee members when he said that "It was fun, one sensed there were groundbreaking elements to it", but he also described it as "an informal, rather agreeable club".[17] There were no terms of reference, formal rules for composition or rotation of membership; to a large extent, the effectiveness of the Committee relied on the personalities of its members, not least Michael Furmston's inimitable style.

# THREE

# Advisory to independent: a missed opportunity

The status of the Committee evolved over many years as the formalisation of the governance of medical research expanded locally, nationally and internationally. Whatever its official status, the Committee was unyielding in its determination to protect the Study participants and prevent the Study and University from disrepute. The necessity to submit ALSPAC studies to further ethical approvals from the local National Health Service (NHS) Research Ethics Committees (RECs), after the thorough and informed scrutiny of the ALSPAC Committee was debatable. The bureaucracy also became increasingly burdensome to many medical research studies, not just ALSPAC. When the ALSPAC Committee was registered as an Independent Review Board in the US, which provided internationally recognised independent status, dual approval by the NHS could have been revised. This would have been a sensible and timely change as it happened to coincide with the ALSPAC Committee being formally incorporated into the University of Bristol's governance structure.

The ALSPAC Ethics and Law Committee's initial status as an advisory committee to Jean Golding was confirmed by David Baum's reassuring letter to the Chair of one of the NHS District Ethics Research Committees in January 1991, nine months after the establishment of the ALSPAC Committee:

The ALSPAC Sub-Committee that advises on ethical and legal matters relating to the ALSPAC studies does *not* in any way serve as an alternative to the District Ethics Research Committee. It serves instead as a discussion group on the difficult and in many ways new problems that arise in relation to a study programme of the ALSPAC magnitude. (David Baum, letter to Denis Savage, January 1991)

The Government guidelines published only 10 days before this letter stated: 'An LREC [Local Research Ethics Committee] must be consulted about any research proposal involving: NHS patients (i.e. subjects recruited by virtue of their past or present treatment by the NHS) ... the use of, or potential access to, NHS premises or facilities.'[1] The recruitment procedure for some, but not all, ALSPAC participants did indeed involve the NHS, both staff and premises, as seen in Box 2.[2] Therefore, there was no question of the necessity of NHS Ethics Committees' approvals at the beginning of the Study but continuing approval for research carried out by ALSPAC over the years was less clear. From the beginning, the ALSPAC Ethics and Law Committee provided thorough ethical scrutiny of ALSPAC as a whole, by lawyers and other appropriate professionals, while universities and the NHS took many years to establish effective governance, particularly for longitudinal epidemiological studies such as ALSPAC. Gordon Stirrat's view was that "we should try to get away from putting things to the LRECs when it was possible. When we were not dealing directly with individuals as patients, we had no need to statutorily; therefore, we shouldn't do so".[3] This view was shared by most of the Committee as not only did ALSPAC make no demands on NHS resources once it was up and running, but also many of the issues being considered by the ALSPAC Committee were of a non-medical nature and beyond the scope of the LRECs. As Elizabeth Mumford described:

"There was, I think, a slight sense of resentment that we had to go there [to the REC] as well as have our own [Ethics Committee]. The feeling was, 'We are doing this, we are doing this really well. Why should we have to send it away to somebody else who doesn't know the Study as well, who is only looking at one little tiny piece of it?'." (Elizabeth Mumford, Oral History Interview, 2013)

---

### Box 2: Enrolment – ALSPAC protocol, seventh edition

Work prior to the start of enrolment in September 1990 had involved meetings with midwives and discussion with groups representing general practitioners as well as detailed discussion with obstetricians in the area. A variety of methods were used to engage the interest of eligible pregnant mothers:

- Posters were printed for display in a variety of different places – including chemist shops, libraries, mother and toddler groups, pre-school playgroups, general practitioner waiting-rooms, antenatal clinics and any other area where a mother was likely to be in early pregnancy.
- The poster displayed the logo of the study 'Children of the Nineties' and asked interested pregnant mothers to get in touch with the study team.
- ALSPAC staff approached eligible mothers when they attended for routine ultrasound examinations.
- The hospitals sent information [about the study] to the mothers with their booking information.
- The local community midwives when interviewing the mother for the first time discussed the study with her and gave her a card with which to send for further details.
- There was considerable local and national coverage in the press, radio and television.
- After delivery, ALSPAC staff approached eligible but non-enrolled mothers whilst they were in the maternity hospital.

---

Perhaps indicative of the informality of the Committee's working processes, it was known by a variety of names throughout its existence: Ethics Committee[4]; Ethics and Law Advisory Committee[5]; Ethics and Law Sub-Committee[6]; Ethics and Law Committee[7]; and Law and Ethics Committee[8]. This appeared to be common practice; all three local NHS RECs referred to themselves differently at least twice between 1990 and 1992.[9] More recently, ALSPAC's local REC has changed its name four times in four years[10] – South West Central Bristol REC, South West 3 REC, North Somerset and South Bristol REC, and Central and South Bristol REC – but this is due to intense bureaucratic activity, quite the opposite of the informality of the early years of these committees.

After the first few meetings of the Committee, Jean Golding, not Michael Furmston, set the Committee agendas.[11] The first meetings had been taken up with formulating the ground rules on confidentiality and consent, as proposed by Michael Furmston, but it was then necessary to respond to Jean Golding's need for advice on the materials to be sent to participants. This included the initial information brochure and first questionnaires, one of which contained sensitive questions about sexual abuse in childhood. It made sense, as an advisory committee, for Jean Golding to set out the matters on which she needed advice. It was taken on trust that she would present the Committee with all relevant concerns and act on the advice given but, as Gordon Stirrat commented, "We wouldn't have that trust nowadays, we wouldn't be allowed to do that".[12] Similarly, Richard Ashcroft stated that "I don't think it ever occurred to me that there would be something she would be keeping from us…. When you meet her you quickly form the impression of enormous integrity".[13]

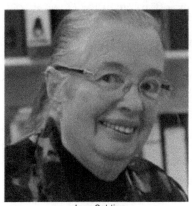

Jean Golding
Source: Bristol Culture

Jean Golding described how she set the agendas:

> "Basically, I think I took everything ... so things like new questionnaires were taken there, how we approached different aspects of contact with pregnant mothers, what we should do about refusals and the whole business of protection of the children was very important but also the protection of the Study from disrepute. So, all of that came into play, so I don't think there was much I didn't present to the Committee, which was why it was meeting so often." (Jean Golding, Oral History Interview, 2012)

Protecting the Study from disrepute was integral to the Committee's deliberations although rarely described in those terms. This was an important ethical matter as should the Study be publically declared or insinuated to be disreputable, participants would be likely to withdraw from the Study and the science would be devalued along with the data already contributed by all Study participants. Fewer participants would reduce the power of the statistical analyses as the vital longitudinal nature of the data from those participants would be limited. For the same reasons, the Committee took into consideration the likelihood of attrition rates being affected when reviewing aspects of the Study.

The initial advisory nature of the Committee was mentioned by nearly all the Committee members when interviewed: "We started as an informal, rather agreeable club helping Jean do her research" stated Tim Chambers when interviewed.[14] Similarly, Michael Furmston thought that "It [ALSPAC] is a massive contribution she [Jean Golding] has made ... everybody else was simply helping her really. Some of us helped quite well I think".[15] Richard Ashcroft elaborated:

> "So, Jean definitely led but she wasn't in the Chair and she was very clear about needing the advice of the Committee and wanting to get the best advice that she could get and she would respond to that advice positively. You never had a sense with her that she didn't like the advice she was getting and she would

just go somewhere else until she got the advice she wanted. She took the Committee very seriously." (Richard Ashcroft, Oral History Interview, 2013)

In 1997, the status of the Committee as advisory was once again confirmed when one member of the Committee raised the question of the relationship between the ALSPAC Committee and that of the LRECs. Was the Committee ultimately responsible for the ethical conduct of the Study, or had it responsibility as part of a chain, or was its responsibility merely to point out areas of concern, with final decision-making in the hands of the LRECs? That the question was asked at all indicates some confusion as to the status of the Committee. The Committee agreed that it was an advisory committee and that ultimate responsibility for decisions lay in the hands of the LRECs,[16] who seemed content at this time with the relatively informal system that had evolved and the ALSPAC updates that they received from Jean Golding.

For the LRECs to be considered to have ultimate responsibility for decisions was odd as they did not review the postal questionnaires, had only partial knowledge of the measurements that were carried out during the research (Children in Focus) clinics and, similarly, did not have comprehensive knowledge of all the other ALSPAC activities, such as home visits by the 'interviewing team' (for participants needing help with completing questionnaires). This lack of comprehensive review by the LRECs was of importance when considering ethical approvals of the many ALSPAC studies that involved secondary analysis only. ALSPAC was designed as a resource for the scientific community and encouraged local, national and international collaboration from 'scientists with bona fide projects of high scientific probity who have promised to abide by the study rules'.[17] Many collaborators' projects were concerned only with secondary analysis; they were not involved in the design or implementation of the data collection. The ALSPAC Ethics and Law Committee did not review these many requests to use data for secondary analyses as these were reviewed by the ALSPAC Scientific Advisory Committee, Genetics Advisory Committee or other ALSPAC advisory committees. Michael Furmston, as Chair of the ALSPAC Ethics and Law Committee, provided a standard letter for these collaborators stating that the Committee had reviewed *all primary* data collections. This statement seemed to satisfy the funding bodies or whoever else needed evidence that the data had been ethically collected, stored and used. This assurance would not have been possible for the LRECs as they had not reviewed in detail all of ALSPAC's many data collections.

Although the intention was for the ALSPAC Committee to review all primary data collections, a few sub-studies did not get ethical review. In February 1999, Jean Golding presented the Committee with an update of ALSPAC sub-studies.[18] There were 18 sub-studies included on the list, of which the Committee had previously been informed of 10. Many of these were not reviewed in detail and there were other sub-studies not included on the list of which the Committee were unaware. It appears that these were overlooked rather than the result of deliberate avoidance (as will be seen in Chapter Thirteen); ethical review was not, as yet, firmly established as part of the research process.

Many collaborators conducted sub-studies that did involve the collection of new or primary data. These studies recruited their participants through ALSPAC and not through the NHS and therefore did not conform to any of the stipulations requiring LREC approval. These new data would then be added to the ALSPAC database and become part of the main ALSPAC resource. Some sub-study collaborators had to gain ethical approval from their own institutions[19] and queried the necessity to seek yet further approval from other probably less qualified committees such as the LRECs. Yet, other collaborating social scientists, including Richard Ashcroft, who resigned from the ALSPAC Committee due to a conflict of interest when he was about to conduct a study on participants' perceptions of their ethical protection, believed that there was no statutory requirement to obtain ethical approval for social research projects (Kent et al, 2002). He and the other Study investigators nevertheless gained ethical approval from a local NHS REC as they felt that this was needed for the satisfactory protection of their participants.

Only one of ALSPAC's many collaborators disputed the necessity for review by the ALSPAC Ethics and Law Committee. This collaborator questioned the ALSPAC Committee's authority to decide whether analyses of cord blood could proceed as ethical approval had been obtained from the LREC. The LREC had confirmed that routine clinical specimens that would normally be discarded could be available for other usage as long as they were anonymised. This was not as stringent as ALSPAC's guarantee to participants that no bio-sample analyses would take place without written consent. As the results of the laboratory analyses would eventually be linked to ALSPAC data, the Committee felt that the ALSPAC policy should apply even though the collaborator, who wanted these analyses conducted as a matter of urgency, was willing to wait for explicit consent before linkage took place.[20]

## Institutional Review Board status

By 2002, the University of Bristol's top-level Ethics of Research Committee had been established and this Committee's oversight of the ALSPAC Ethics and Law Committee was confirmed when the ALSPAC Committee was registered as an Institutional Review Board (IRB) with the US Office of Human Research Protections.[21] Surprisingly, the registration took place without formal consultation with the Committee. One of ALSPAC's collaborators thought that it would be useful as he was funded by an institution in the US and confirmation of IRB approval was necessary for this funding. This registration formally recognised the ability of the ALSPAC Committee to provide appropriate independent ethical review. This was useful for ALSPAC's many collaborators from the US or others funded by US bodies, who frequently needed evidence that suitable review had taken place and IRB approval fulfilled the necessary official requirements. More importantly, this change in status for the ALSPAC Committee, now recognised as an independent committee and incorporated into the University's governance structure, was a missed opportunity for the Committee. To be confirmed as an internationally recognised independent committee and no longer merely advisory could have been the opportunity to discard the burdensome LREC approvals. Unfortunately, the Committee was not made aware of this change in status and therefore not able to consider the implications. Even if the ALSPAC Committee had recognised and taken this opportunity, it would have been a brief respite as in 2011, after Michael Furmston and Jean Golding had retired, the Department of Health stipulated that all studies involving the collection of bio-samples must have local NHS REC approval.[22]

The evolving importance and formalisation of the ethics of research, both within the university and in the NHS from 1990 when the Committee was set up, was bound to impact on the ALSPAC Ethics and Law Committee eventually. The opportunity to escape the increasingly bureaucratic LREC approvals, as detailed in the next chapter, was missed when its independent status as an IRB was authorised.

# FOUR

# Bureaucratic battles: liaison with Local Research Ethics Committees

Any research that involved National Health Service (NHS) resources required Local Research Ethics Committee (LREC) approval but most of ALSPAC's research had no impact on these resources. LREC approvals could have provided an extra level of protection for the Study participants but the LRECs seemed to be overwhelmed with the increasing amount of paperwork that they requested. It is well documented that their own bureaucratic processes became unethically onerous around the beginning of the millennium. At this time, ALSPAC was subject to untimely and inconsistent decisions by the LRECs, resulting in, for example, unnecessary (and costly) delays to the start of one clinic and prohibiting the use of genetic material from another. Throughout this period, the ALSPAC Ethics and Law Committee provided comprehensive ethical protection for the Study participants while endeavouring to negotiate a pragmatic working relationship with these local committees.

The ALSPAC catchment area covered three District Health Authorities, each with its own LREC: Bristol & Weston, Southmead and Frenchay. During the planning and piloting of ALSPAC, David Baum had written to the Chairs of these committees outlining the Study[1] and this was followed by official application forms for ethical approval from Jean Golding.[2] In those days (1989), the forms were brief (two to four sides), designed with clinical trials in mind and mostly concerned with the use of drugs or radioactive materials. These LRECs gave their approval to the Study with only a few concerns: the use of NHS staff during recruitment and the sensitive handling of mothers who suffered stillbirths or miscarriages. They did request to see recruitment materials and questionnaires and wanted confirmation that the ALSPAC Ethics and Law Committee was an advisory committee only and not an alternative to the LRECs.

For many years, Jean Golding supplied the LRECs with considerable amounts of information without having to formally seek further ethical approval. During 1990, she sent the initial participant information sheets, letters and first questionnaires, followed in 1991 by 12 more questionnaires, including those to be sent to women who had miscarried, and the first 'Children of the Nineties' birthday card and newsletters. In 1992, a general update was sent informing the LRECs of: an extension to the enrolment dates; a list of bio-samples that would be analysed (only with written consent); the intention to look at medical records, including of the eligible mothers who had not enrolled (the latter not approved by one committee and abandoned); and the plan for a variety of sub-studies. Ethical approval of sub-studies was far from consistent. Some submitted their own separate applications to the LRECs but this was often only to one of the committees, for example, 'Indoor air pollution and lower respiratory illness in infancy'[3] or 'A population based study of neonatal cerebral ultrasound in the prediction of later impairment'[4] (which was approved but not implemented as financial support was not forthcoming).

The application for the first ALSPAC research clinics, submitted to all three LRECs, entitled 'Is screening for anaemia in the first two years of life worthwhile?', contained the barest of details:

> A 10% sample of the ALSPAC study will be asked to take part in this. They will be sent a letter which asked them to come to a clinic to be held at 6, 12 and 18 months of age. At the clinic the children will be given cognitive function tests, growth will be measured accurately and a 3-day dietary diary will be

administered to the mother. A heel prick will be used to take a small sample of blood from the baby provided the mother is happy with this. (Submission for ethical approval, Bristol and Weston LREC, April 1992)

This was the application for what was to become an exceptionally important ALSPAC sub-study, 'Children in Focus' (initially called 'The 10% club'). These children, numbering approximately 1,400, were invited to attend initially at the age of four months and then nine more times in their first five years. The measurements in these clinics ranged far wider than first envisaged in the infant anaemia study and included measurements of blood pressure, lung function, fitness, skin observations, allergy tests, dental observations and vision, hearing and language assessments, as well as environmental measures in the families' homes and a parenting measure. These changes were not reviewed and approved by the LRECs prospectively.

Ethical approval from the LRECs continued to be informal and not entirely consistent for many years. Jean Golding regarded sending information about the Study as "a courtesy".[5] In 1993, she sent a report on the 'Survey Development and Protocol' with a covering letter that stated: 'I trust that the study as set out in this document continues to meet with your approval'.[6] Some extra information concerning change in blood-sampling methods was sent in 1994 and then similar survey reports were again sent in 1995 and 1997. Mostly, there was little response to these reports although there was considerable concern from the Chair of one committee about allergy (skin prick) tests at the final 'Children in Focus' clinic. Included in the correspondence about this issue was the request that a new proposal was submitted as it was in question 'whether this additional test can be regarded as an extension of the original proposal to administer questions'.[7] A proposal was duly submitted and approved 'with the proviso that the information sheet states that you are looking at gene markers'.[8] This was not the case and suggests that the LREC had not grasped the issues. The other two committees had no concerns, although the status of the approval was in question as the letter from one committee Secretary stated that the Chair was 'happy for you to continue the study in this way. If however you require formal approval, perhaps you would let me know'.[9] Approval from the LRECs appeared to be optional; as Tim Chambers reflected, "they [the LRECs] were feeling their way".[10]

The LRECs were aware that ALSPAC had its own ethics advisory committee as this was frequently mentioned in correspondence. It can be assumed that the LRECs were also aware of the nature of the work of the ALSPAC Committee, in that the Committee formulated ethical principles in the process of detailed and comprehensive review of all aspects of the Study.

By 1998, the planning for 'Focus at 7', the first half-day research clinic for all Study children (numbering over 8,000) was well underway. The ALSPAC Committee reviewed in detail the considerable number of relevant documents: protocols, invitation letters, participant information sheets, consent forms and so on. Policies such as divulging individual results were developed and clarified[11] before a full application was subsequently submitted to the four LRECs (the original three had become four). This would be the case annually until 2004, when the regulations changed allowing the necessity for only one LREC application. By this time, the relationship between the ALSPAC Committee and the LRECs had deteriorated. As Gordon Stirrat recalled:

"The relationship with the Local Research Ethics Committees, as they were, was really problematical and my recollection was that we decided, well, we probably didn't need to go to them for most of the things.... But, regrettably, my view of the Local Research Ethics Committees was not high. I didn't think the understanding, the quality of the people, some were good in their own fields but their understanding of ethics of research was partial ... they really hadn't a proper training.... They had *no idea at all* what was involved in an epidemiological longitudinal study." (Gordon Stirrat, Oral History Interview, 2013)

Towards the end of the 1990s, the work involved was substantial not only for the LREC members and administrators, but also for the NHS Trust Research and Development Departments, from whom approval was also necessary. One Trust required yet further review by a Paediatric Research & Development Peer Support Group. Considering the amount of work involved in reviewing aspects of the Study such as the research clinics, which had no impact on NHS resources, it is surprising that the LRECs were willing to undertake this work. In fact, for one LREC, it was quite the opposite; the review of an ALSPAC sub-study by another university's Faculty Ethics Committee was not considered adequate and a formal LREC submission was requested.[12]

It is clear that any research that did involve NHS premises, staff or other resources required LREC approval but this was not the case for the vast majority of ALSPAC's research. Apart from the expense involved in complying with the bureaucratic demands of LRECs, these demands were being questioned by many as being so extreme as to be unethical (Glasziou and Chalmers, 2004; Al-Shahi, 2005). The LRECs relevant to ALSPAC seemed to be overwhelmed with the paperwork. For example, on one occasion, there was baffling inconsistency of approvals by one LREC, which, when the discrepancy was pointed out, demonstrated determined inflexibility, as did the governing body, the Central Office for Research Ethics Committees (COREC). ALSPAC had submitted *identical* paperwork for the collection of blood samples from parents attending ALSPAC clinics with their children; one set of paperwork was submitted as an amendment to an already established clinic, the other as part of a new application for the next annual clinic. The paperwork for both submissions was reviewed at the *same LREC meeting* but, astonishingly, the amendment was approved with no ethical concerns while the same procedure for the new clinic was rejected. The reasons for the objection were equally baffling and showed little knowledge, not only of ALSPAC's methodology, but also of their previous (or, in this case, simultaneous) approvals for identical procedures. The LREC members apparently felt '... that any proposed research involving this collection [of] DNA and Cell lines ... should be subject to further ethical review by the Research

Ethics Committee'.[13] This would mean that every new analysis of these samples would require a new submission to the LRECs. Jean Golding did not point out at this stage the inconsistency between approvals, but explained ALSPAC processes:

> This request is not really feasible with this type of large, longitudinal, epidemiological study. Genotyping is carried out for certain collaborators, usually with a candidate gene in mind, after peer review and ethical approval from their institutions and the funding bodies. As with all data, secondary analyses will be conducted for years to come depending on developments and hypotheses generated within the scientific community. Some of the results of this analysis will be published, much won't as it will not be relevant to the papers which are written. All analyses are only carried out after strict anonymisation (reversible as explained in the COREC form, Part B, Section 5) and we only allow analyses using genotype results by our own statisticians or occasionally on in-house stand-alone computers. We have been abstracting DNA from the cohort for seven years on this understanding with no objection from the cohort and with approval from the LRECs. (Letter to LREC Chair from Jean Golding, December 2004)

The restriction on this use of the ALSPAC genetic resource had severe consequences. While Jean Golding and Michael Furmston tried to persuade the LRECs to change their mind, taking blood from parents and children at this clinic had to be delayed. When it became obvious that the LREC would not see sense, ALSPAC agreed to their conditions so that they could collect and store blood and then attempt to overturn the decision at a later date. Eventually, after three years, the LREC decision was overturned with considerable effort from Professor George Davey Smith, who had, by then, succeeded Jean Golding as Director of ALSPAC.[14]

This was one of an extensive list of clashes with the LRECs that seemed to climax in 2004.[15] It is not possible to determine how

Michael Furmston's unusual approach was received by the Chair of an LREC at this time. One letter started 'Let me speak in a frank and comradely fashion as Breznev said to Dubcek or vice versa' but the substance of his correspondence was far from flippant, as can be seen.[16]

> ... the current process of gaining ethical approval from your committee does not accommodate the complexities of a large, well-established, longitudinal cohort such as ALSPAC. As you know, this will be the seventh annual ALSPAC clinic involving over one hundred staff and thousands of parents and children; we are obviously reluctant to postpone the start unless there are grave ethical concerns that need to be addressed.

He went on:

> Let me come to the question of non-administrative amendments. You say in the fifth paragraph of your letter 'The committee would like to express its concern that ALSPAC, with its wealth of research experience, appears reluctant to submit the relevant documentation for ethics approval, and we would welcome a commitment to do so in the future.' Your committee must of course be aware that the ethical aspects of all these changes will continue to be considered by the ALSPAC Law & Ethics committee. It is not a question therefore of considering ethics approval but of how much paper we should send in your direction. It may well be that the members of your committee feel much more able to deal with the ethical problems than my committee but this view is not shared by my committee members. Of course, neither of us is wholly dispassionate in this respect. The problem I was trying to address in my previous letter was not so much ethics as timetable. Imagine the captain of a super-tanker who had to steer according to the guidance of your committee. What we wanted to do was to try to devise a working scheme, which would fit into the timetable requirements to which you are required to work.

A further issue involved a sub-study that had already been reviewed and approved by the collaborators' own institution as well as the ALSPAC Committee:

> Much of the research being done by ALSPAC could be done by social scientists who would not go near your committee and would indeed be astonished that your committee members would have any particular expertise in the sort of work they are doing. If push comes to shove we may have to open up this can of worms but for the moment I am mindful of Pandora. As far as [this] … study is concerned, it has already been rigorously scrutinised by two committees and I was and still am anxious to avoid excessive delay and the generation of yet more paper.

As Gordon Stirrat related:

> "Michael didn't suffer fools gladly…. He went to see an Ethics Committee. I don't think he helped by telling them exactly what he thought of them. Now, he had justification for doing so, but diplomatically it was not the thing to do and that caused a rift."[17]

During the 1990s and 2000s, not only the understanding of the ethics of research, but also the processes involved to ensure the protection of research participants, underwent major developments. During this time, the LRECs' requirements evolved from minimal retrospective information to demands for unmanageable quantities of documentation (both paper and electronic), resulting in untimely and inconsistent decisions. In parallel, the University was developing its own structures for understanding and dealing with ethical issues in research, although these did not impact on ALSPAC much during Jean Golding's and Michael Furmston's era. Throughout this period, the ALSPAC Ethics and Law Committee provided relative consistency and stability while trying to negotiate a pragmatic working relationship with the LRECs. It was almost certainly unique for the LRECs to have to accommodate the judgements of another better-qualified committee and, as Elizabeth Mumford understated, this created "a slightly uneasy relationship".[18]

# Part Two
# Policy development:
# a case of case law

# FIVE

# Confidentiality and anonymity: a rod for their own backs

The guarantee to Study participants that their data would be anonymised, not just kept confidential, produced some highly innovative policies, such as the 'Ethical Divide'. Although this enabled much of ALSPAC's work to be carried out with robust protection of participants' anonymity, issues continually arose requiring further thought and adjustment to the policies. Data access, especially issues of deductive disclosure and the misuse of data, were early concerns of the Committee. These became particularly problematic as time went on as there was increasing pressure by funding and government bodies to allow greater access to publicly funded data sets.

As David Baum stated when he first proposed an ALSPAC Ethics Committee, 'establishing the absolute principle of non-attributability'[1] was considered of the utmost importance from the Study's inception. Aspects of this principle and the wide-ranging implications for the infrastructure and running of the Study were discussed by the Committee throughout its existence. At the very first meeting in April 1990, Michael Furmston suggested that 'Confidentiality' was one of the two 'general issues requiring most careful consideration' by the Committee (the other being 'Consent'). From this first discussion, the Committee returned to the theme time and time again, and strategies emerged. Participants' trust was considered essential if they were to answer questions honestly and supply the Study with sensitive information over many years. The importance of storing, processing and analysing data anonymously was considered of particular importance in a local study such as ALSPAC, where many staff knew participants personally and several staff were also members of the Cohort. Guarantees were made to the participants in the initial information leaflet that they were sent: 'A very complicated set of procedures will ensure that no one will be able to link the information that you give us with your name'.[2] In 1993, David Baum stated that this phrase 'did not have to mean that it would be physically impossible to do so but could also indicate simply that no one would be allowed to do so'.[3] However, even this interpretation of the guarantee could not be adhered to absolutely without hampering bona fide research, such as the selection of cases and controls for sub-studies. Although the leaflet had been reviewed and approved by the Committee, Elizabeth Mumford held that this phrase 'came back again and again to haunt us' (Overy et al, 2012, p 73) as it impacted on so many other ethical issues: child protection; the disclosure of individuals' results; requests for help or other comments on questionnaires; and linkages to third-party data.

## The 'Ethical Divide'

Details concerning anonymity were available on request for Study participants in a letter (see Appendix 3), which described what came to be known by ALSPAC staff as the 'Ethical Divide'. This was the process of keeping data anonymous. All ALSPAC staff were divided into two groups: 'administrative' staff and 'research' staff. The 'administrative' staff were allowed access to names and addresses, and for some teams, this had to include the limited data sets that they were collecting (for example data abstracted from hospital records or face-to-face measurements taken at the clinics) but they were unable to link to data sets from other sources. The 'research' staff, most of whom were statisticians, could link data sets from any sources but were prohibited from accessing names and addresses or other personal identifiers. Gordon Stirrat described this as the "golden rule: the policy by which we quarantined the data so that those who were analysing it and those who were collecting it couldn't contaminate one another".[4] This system, in itself, could not guarantee complete security as it was possible for someone with access to the research database to identify individuals with only a very few pieces of information if they wished to do so, for example, age of mother, number of children, occupation, type of housing or height. This is now known as 'deductive disclosure'. All staff were required to sign a confidentiality form annually and every effort was made to embed a culture of absolute respect for the guarantees given to participants concerning their data but, ultimately, the prevention of deductive disclosure came down to the integrity of the staff. As time went on, collaborators or ALSPAC staff who both collected data and needed to analyse them using links to other data sets had to be accommodated. They were not allowed the central ALSPAC linkage number and were provided with only the specific data sets necessary for their research. There were also circumstances when it was necessary to cross the administration–research divide, not only when selecting participants for sub-studies from questionnaire answers, but also, for example, when identifying participants if they had withdrawn their consent for the use of their bio-samples. There were a limited number of named individuals permitted to do this, which, for many years, consisted of the ALSPAC computing manager and his assistant only.[5]

## The '500 rule'

By 1991, a number of collaborators were interested in carrying out studies on particular subgroups of children, for example, children with severe speech impediments. Selection could be made from the mothers' questionnaire answers but if the policy of not linking data to names was observed, further study of these individuals would not be possible. The Committee decided that controls should be selected and any fieldworkers meeting the Study participants would be blind to the individuals' status (that is case or control).[6] So, the policy on confidentiality began to evolve. In 1993, when the problem arose again, the Committee spent three meetings struggling with the issue,[7] in particular, the possibility of researchers being interested in a very small number of cases. This was when the '500 rule' was established, which recommended that at least one control per case was selected with the total selected numbering at least 500; this arbitrary figure was considered adequate to protect confidentiality. In 1999, the (unwritten) rule was amended when a collaborator asked to conduct in-depth interviews with 300 girls (selected for high and low risk of engaging in anti-social behaviour). Conducting more than 300 interviews was not feasible due to limitations in funding. The Committee decided that the 500 rule could be waived but only with specific project approval by the Committee. To waive an ethical rule due to financial considerations might be considered unprincipled but this was a pragmatic response that enabled the research to go ahead without, so the Committee believed, compromising the guarantee of anonymity given to the participants. It could be considered unethical to prevent important research being carried out by rigidly adhering to the arbitrary figure of 500. Other requests to waive ALSPAC's ethical policies for financial reasons were not necessarily granted. One request that was denied was for the analysis of bio-samples without participant consent on the grounds that the enforced delay while consent was sought would threaten the job of a research assistant as there was not enough money to cover their salary.

## Questionnaires

Prior to the first questionnaires being sent to participating mothers, the Committee discussed a variety of issues concerning young mothers (both under 16 and under 18), including:

> ... the practical matter of sending questionnaires to a home where it is possible that some or all family members are unaware of the girl's pregnancy, or where the girl has not yet accepted the fact that she is pregnant or decided whether or not to keep the baby (both situations are prevalent among young mothers). (Appendix 4, 'Young mothers', by Elizabeth Mumford, submitted to Committee, November 1990)

The Committee pragmatically suggested that all questionnaires should initially be sent in 'innocuous-looking envelopes with no ALSPAC logo'.[8]

The guarantee not to link names with data again became an issue when participants added comments to their questionnaires anticipating a reply. ALSPAC's solution to this was to ask participants to sign their comments if they wanted a reply. All self-completion questionnaires stated 'N.B. Please remember we cannot reply to any comment unless you sign it'. In 2003, the Family Liaison Manger asked the Committee for clarification concerning unsigned comments on returned questionnaires. As documented in the minutes:

> Linking of unsigned information to the study family was breaking the ALSPAC rules of confidentiality but in certain exceptional circumstances, e.g. 'partner has died', the information was acted on to make sure no further questionnaires were sent out. The committee agreed that common sense should be applied to information detailing change of circumstances. (Committee minutes, December 2003)

A protocol was drafted that was approved by the Committee at their next meeting.[9] The wording on the back of the questionnaires was also changed very slightly at the recommendation of the Committee: 'Please remember we can't reply to comments in this space unless you sign your full name'. As can be seen in Chapter Ten, this facet of the confidentiality guarantee created difficult decisions for the Committee, which spent much time over the years considering individual cases, which were not always resolved consistently.

## Text data

In 2002, another related confidentiality issue came to the Committee's attention: the processing of text data (that is hand-written comments) from self-completion questionnaires. These data (such as medications, types of accident, reasons for hospital admissions) were keyed into a database without names attached. This did not necessarily make these data anonymous as dates or uncommon events made the data easily identifiable. It was recommended that names, places of residence and dates were removed, although the Committee allowed Jean Golding to use her judgement if collaborators needed to know, for example, places of residence in relation to certain diseases.[10]

## Genetic data

Analysis of genetic data and the protection of participants' anonymity was a concern that was resolved before ever being brought before the Committee. Genotyping was not carried out by ALSPAC as there were many laboratories, including commercial ones, better equipped to do this efficiently, which constantly updated their equipment and expertise as technology improved. Researchers receiving DNA for genotyping were required to return genotypes to ALSPAC for linkage to other data. They were not permitted to carry out further genotyping without permission from ALSPAC's Genetic Advisory Committee and had to return remaining DNA once genotyping was complete. These genotypic data were returned to ALSPAC (very occasionally along with bio-sample residue) but, from the first analyses of genetic data in 1997, were only linked to other ALSPAC data by ALSPAC statisticians who conducted the genetic analyses. Collaborators needing genetic analyses could either instruct the ALSPAC statisticians to do this or conduct the analyses themselves working on stand-alone machines within ALSPAC with the assistance of ALSPAC statisticians. This prevented them from being able to link to any other ALSPAC data sets without authorisation.

## Data access

Access to ALSPAC data, even in anonymised form, was a concern for the Committee not just due to the risk of deductive disclosure, but also as it was considered possible for data to be misused if analysed and published irresponsibly, for example, if genes were analysed in relation to race for political, not scientific, reasons. The Committee regarded it as their duty to prevent such misuse while recognising that it was vital that responsible collaborators were encouraged to access data and allowed to do so with the minimum of difficulties. Conditions for collaboration evolved from "gentlemanly guidelines"[11] mostly concerned with the return of data to ALSPAC to more formal 'Conditions for collaboration' reviewed by the Committee in 1996.[12] These covered: scientific approval; funding; ethical approval; additional data collection; data access and utilisation; publications; and accountability.

As time went on, there was increasing pressure by funding and government bodies to allow greater access to publicly funded data sets. Under close supervision by the Committee, who were concerned about breaches in anonymity and misuse of data, and after lengthy discussion in many meetings during 2005, ALSPAC deposited selected data sets with the UK Data Archive.[13] This resource, supported by the Economic & Social Research Council, provides access for secondary analysis of large data sets to researchers and other academics mostly in the fields of economics and other social sciences.

The guarantee of anonymity was fundamental to ALSPAC's design but it did generate complexities not anticipated at the beginning of the Study. The prevention of Study participants being identified by staff or collaborators was especially important in such a localised study. Irreversible anonymisation is not possible in longitudinal studies such as ALSPAC as the linking of sequential data from individuals is integral to the methodology. The highly innovative 'Ethical Divide' enabled much of ALSPAC's work to be carried out with satisfactory protection of participants but issues arose repeatedly over the years, requiring further thought and adjustment to the policies. Constant vigilance was essential as this guarantee impacted on so many aspects of the Study, and the Committee had to spend much of its time finding solutions that would preserve the guarantee.

# SIX

# Informed consent:
# too much information

The complexities and practical considerations of aspects of consent (such as written, implied, informed, withdrawal, dual [parent and child], sole [child only] or assent) that covered all the many measures collected by ALSPAC, comprised much of the Committee's workload throughout its existence. Of particular importance and originality, which was considered highly controversial at the time, was the strategy of 'broad' consent for the use of genetic material. This allowed for unspecified future research, not only on abstracted DNA, but also on 'immortalised' cell lines, which could be used to make more DNA far into the future. Participants' trust in the investigators was recognised as crucial and, to this end, honest explanation of the research was necessary. Yet, too much information could be discouraging and balance in this respect was always the Committee's aim.

The principle of informed consent was one of the fundamentals of the Ethics Committee's 'constitution', as termed by Elizabeth Mumford. At the very first Committee meeting, Michael Furmston outlined what he felt were the central questions:

1. From whom should consent be sought? The mother? Her partner? Anyone else?

2. To what should consent be given? General participation in the Study? The use of biological samples?
3. By what process should consent be obtained? 'Opting in' versus 'opting out'. Will a written form suffice? How much explanation is necessary? (Committee minutes, April 1990)

## From whom?

### Mothers

Although the Committee's minutes state 'Naturally the mother should be asked to give consent to her own participation in the study',[1] when the process of enrolment was described by Professor Golding at the same meeting, it was agreed that a consent form as such was not necessary:

Dr Golding explained that, as soon as a pregnancy became known to medical personnel, the doctor or midwife concerned would send the name of the pregnant woman to ALSPAC. A leaflet would then be sent to the mother, describing the project, and briefly stating what would take place (questionnaires, tissue samples). No actual 'consent form' was envisaged. Consent would be 'implied' if the parents did not specifically refuse to participate. (Committee minutes, May 1990)

It is doubtful that it would be acceptable now to enrol participants without written consent, although whether this would comprise a risk to patients is dubious. The return of self-completion questionnaires continues to be considered acceptable as 'implied consent'. At that time, self-completion questionnaires and biological samples were the only suggested methods of data collection for ALSPAC, with written consent strictly observed before any analyses of biological samples.

## Mothers' partners

The Study design included mothers' partners, whether they were the biological father or not, as Jean Golding recognised that their social influences were as important as the biological influences on the Study child. This was one of several unique features of ALSPAC. A leaflet circulated to potential funders and collaborators in 1989 outlining the Study stated that 'it will be the first geographically-based population study involving the personalities, behaviour and attitudes of both mother and father'.[2] The Committee therefore agreed that the partner would not necessarily be the putative father (that is assumed biological father), but be defined as 'the person who was the mother's partner at the time of first contact and to any subsequent partner who appeared during the course of the study'.[3] This was an important decision, although it created some administrative complications as partners changed over time or questionnaires were written assuming partners were male when some partners were female. The mother was left to decide if she wanted her partner involved in the Study and the final version of the initial leaflet stated:

> If you are living with a husband or partner, we would very much like to include them in the research. Partners can be an important influence on the health and development of a child. If you agree we will give you a questionnaire to pass on to him. His answers will, like yours, be confidential and he will be asked to return his questionnaire directly to us. The decision to include your partner in the study, however will be yours. (Initial information leaflet sent to participants)

## Children

The children's cooperation or assent for any procedure was always paramount but the Committee decided that from the age of 12, their signed consent for biological samples and certain other measurements was necessary along with parental consent. Although probably not legally binding, the Committee felt that this would provide a formal opportunity for the children not only to address any concerns they had to the researchers, but also to be informed of what would happen to their data.[4] At 16 years old, sole consent from the Study child was considered acceptable by the Committee and although the law was not specific about young people with regards to research, this complied with the Family Law Reform Act 1969[5] as regards treatment: those who are 16 years old or above have the same legal ability to consent to any medical, surgical or dental treatment as anyone above 18, without consent from their parent or guardian.

### Adults lacking capacity to consent

During the first year of the Committee meeting, adults considered by the Committee members to be lacking the capacity to consent due to 'mental handicap or mental or physical illness' and 'very young mothers who do not have the maturity to give consent' were considered when Elizabeth Mumford presented a brief document outlining the legal position with these participants:

Presumably, it would still be of interest to have information about such women and this might be provided by their parents, guardians or other family members. The decision about whether a woman was capable of participating would ideally be made by the midwife/G.P. and following this, the questionnaires might be altered to eliminate those things which could not be answered by proxy (e.g. state of mind). (Appendix 4, 'Young mothers', by Elizabeth Mumford, submitted to Committee, November 1990)

The adaption of the questionnaires recommended by Elizabeth Mumford was endorsed by the Committee. The ALSPAC Family Liaison Team, known perhaps confusingly as 'the interviewers' for many years, who kept an ever-changing database of those participants who needed extra help or sensitive handling, administered the questionnaires. This would usually be by conducting a home visit and either administering the questionnaires themselves or ensuring that the parents or guardians were comfortable in doing so, omitting inappropriate questions. It seems that it was simpler to keep this task within the Family Liaison Team without involving GPs or midwives.

## To what and by what process?

### Questionnaires and bio-samples

The Committee decided rapidly that if questionnaires were returned, whether by Study mother, partner or children (who started receiving their own postal questionnaires from the age of five), consent could be implied.[6] In the early 1990s (before the introduction of the Human Tissue Act), there was no legal requirement to obtain informed consent to use biological samples from participants. However, the Committee were keen to ensure that bio-samples were only used with the consent of the mothers. The first bio-samples collected by ALSPAC were collected through the National Health Service (NHS) (for example antenatal blood, cord blood and placentas), with the NHS obtaining consent for therapeutic purposes only. The Committee were clear that this was not adequate for the non-therapeutic research purposes proposed by ALSPAC, so mothers were asked at a later date to sign a consent form to give ALSPAC permission to use them for research.[7] The first biological samples obtained by ALSPAC (not NHS) staff were taken at the Children in Focus clinics. Initially, these were heel-prick samples (at eight, 12 and 18 months old), but subsequently, venous blood samples were taken after the application of anaesthetic cream (EMLA cream). Consent from parents was recorded, although, in the early clinics, this was not in the format recommended nowadays. Nevertheless, ALSPAC was collecting consent from participants long before this became a legal requirement in 2006. The postal collection of the Cohort children's milk teeth was taken as implied consent as parents would not have sent the teeth if they did not agree to their use.

Sampling of fathers' blood was initially considered too sensitive to be acceptable because of potential paternity issues. The issue was discussed in the first year of the Committee's existence at the request of the Steering Committee (identified in the Ethics Committee minutes as the 'Scientific Group'). Although there was 'significant interest in assessing the genetic contribution of the child's father', both Committees expressed concern. The Ethics Committee minutes state:

> There is a significant proportion (not less than 5% and probably between 10–30%) of fathers who raise children not biologically their own. Inevitably some men within that group are not aware that the child is not their own, others would be unwilling to share this information with anyone else, even as part of a confidential study. The mere fact of asking for paternal samples might be seen as threatening and could prompt some mothers to withdraw from the study altogether. Hence, the Committee agreed with the conclusion reached by the Scientific Group, that prudential consideration probably outweighed the scientific merit of the exercise. (Committee minutes, September 1990)

It was not until 1996 that this decision was overturned and the Ethics Committee agreed to the collection of partners' saliva through the post for genetic studies as 'there have been interesting findings lately about patterns of inheritance, suggesting that children inherit things differently from their mothers and their fathers'.[8] The Committee thought that written consent would *not* be necessary 'as there was no bodily intervention being carried out by study personnel'.[9] Although this implied that there could therefore be no legal accusations of battery, it did not comply with the Committee's previous insistence that written consent must be obtained before analysis of any bio-samples. Despite the Committee's recommendation, others in ALSPAC took a more cautious view and written consent forms were included in the postal packs, making it quite clear that the samples were for genetic analyses. This very simple consent form was sent with a brief Question & Answer information sheet (see Boxes 3 and 4), which had been seen and approved by the Committee. This set a remarkable precedent for genetic research on population-based studies like ALSPAC as only very broad or 'blanket consent' was obtained. Any genetic analyses could be conducted without informing the participants of the nature of the research and without obtaining further consent. Although this is now standard practice in genomic research, both at the time and for many years afterwards, it was considered controversial (Caulfield et al, 2003).

## Box 3: Participant information sheet (partner's mouthwash)

### Some questions and answers

*Q: I can understand why you want to study the genes of my child, but why of me and my partner?*
A: You and your partner are also very important to the study because so little is known about the health and well-being of young men and women – and how to improve things for them in the future.

*Q: Surely DNA is only used for looking at criminals or deciding who is the father of a child?*
A: Well, that is certainly what hits the headlines and the DNA can be used for those purposes. That is not the aim of the study though. We are interested in your partner regardless of whether he is the father of the study child or not. Of course we are interested too in the DNA of those partners who are the fathers of the Children of the 90s, as we are interested in the ways in which abilities and healthiness are inherited.

*Q: What are the most exciting questions that you think the DNA will help solve?*
A: The whole question of asthma and allergies. We know that whole families can be affected, but other children, and their parents, can suddenly become allergic or develop asthma out of the blue. But why? Partly it is by contact with something like pets or air pollution, but many people are also in contact with these things and do not develop asthma. The secret lies in finding out what the protective genes are. Discovery of which the protective genes are may show us all how to stop asthma occurring.

## Box 4: Partner mouthwash consent form

Children of the Nineties
24 Tyndall Avenue
Bristol BS8 1TQ

**HUSBAND/PARTNER CONSENT FORM**

**The Genetic Study**

I am happy to give this mouthwash to the Children of the Nineties in order for research to be carried out into the genetic causes of health and illness.

I understand that the results will never be linked to my name or that of any of my family.

Signed.............................................. Date......................

1. FULL NAME (capital letters please)

...................................................................................................

2. Your date of birth

| | | | | | 1 | 9 | | |

3. Your relationship to the study child (please tick one)

Biological father

Male partner

Female partner

*Thank you so much*

**Please put this consent form in the return envelope with the mouthwash.**

By 1999, the Committee reviewed a more extensive information sheet written by Marcus Pembrey for parents who wished to have more information about the genetic aspects of the Study,[10] and by 2001, for the Focus at 9 clinics, information sheets were available for both children and parents.

## How much explanation is necessary?

When the Committee met for only the second time in May 1990, another fundamental of Elizabeth Mumford's 'constitution' was discussed. This concerned information for participants and the minutes state that the 'educative process was the most crucial element in securing a balance between the study's success in maximising both the number of participants and subsequent participant satisfaction'.[11] This may seem beyond the remit of the Committee but maximising participant numbers was crucial for the scientific validity of the Study. If numbers were not adequate, the data given by participants would be wasted and this would be unethical if avoidable. Participant satisfaction also needed to be considered when weighing up the risks and benefits of whatever the participants were being asked to do and could be considered a relevant judgement for the Committee. Although not explicitly stated at that meeting, the Participant Information Sheets (PIS) were also considered an integral part of the process of gaining informed consent. This was quite a new concept and beyond any legal requirement.

The Committee endeavoured to review every consent form and PIS before implementation; during the first 16 years, nearly 200 of these documents came to the Committee. Many aspects had to be considered, from the tone and readability (as the average reading age of the general population was well below that of the researchers who created the documents), to the amount of information given, with special attention as to the age of the participants. Separate information sheets were frequently produced for adults and children. Too much information was considered as detrimental as too little information. In a longitudinal study such as ALSPAC, there was an accumulation of knowledge by the participants over many years and it was thought by the Committee that an excess of information could be discouraging.

## Other aspects of consent

Although Michael Furmston and the Committee focused on consent for questionnaires and biological samples in the early Committee meetings, over the following years, other issues around consent took up much of the Committee's time.

### Withdrawal of consent

Withdrawal of consent had to be considered by the Committee from early on, although, as with other ALSPAC policies, it was not formally documented until long after Jean Golding had retired. In May 1992, the Committee were asked to consider:

> Could the information collected before the women's withdrawal from the study be used?... Mr Hirschmann pointed out that there might be two types of 'drop-outs'; those who were simply tired of participating and those who regretted their choice to take part. Professor Furmston suggested that if there were any specific requests to have material collected in the past destroyed on withdrawal from the study, then such a request ought to be met. (Committee minutes, May 1992)

It is not clear if the 'material' referred to bio-samples or other data. Bio-samples could be and were on occasions destroyed but the withdrawal of information already processed, analysed and published was not possible. The following year, the Committee decided that:

> ... the onus was on the woman to indicate if the withdrawal was intended to be retrospective as well as prospective. However, as a matter of good practice all those who communicated their intention to withdraw personally should be asked whether it

was because of some specific incident or problem. (Committee minutes, August 1993)

It was not suggested that this personal contact would be an opportunity to establish if the withdrawal was for retrospective as well as prospective data, presumably because of the difficulties of withdrawing data from ALSPAC's 'built files' (processed data, including summary statistics). By 2003, Michael Furmston decided that Study children 'should not be able to opt out retrospectively; it was sufficient that consent had been obtained at the time'.[12] Throughout Jean Golding's and Michael Furmston's time on the Committee, requests to withdraw from the Study were dealt with on a case-by-case basis by the Family Liaison Team, with very occasional referral to the Committee. The emphasis was always that 'children wanting to withdraw from the study should not only be enthusiastically thanked for all they had done with emphasis on how important their contribution had been, but also given easy opportunities to re-join if and when they changed their minds'.[13]

### Gift clause

In 2002, Jean Golding had asked 'if a child wanted their samples to be destroyed was ALSPAC obliged to comply?'.[14] Elizabeth Mumford thought that there was no clear answer as to who owned bio-samples and it was suggested by another Committee member (John Henderson) that perhaps the bio-samples could be considered a gift to the researchers. This was not enacted upon at the time. It was not until a Local Research Ethics Committee (LREC) made the same suggestion that a clause was added to the bio-sample consent forms two years after it had first been suggested. This stated, 'I understand that donated blood will be considered a gift but I will have the right to withdraw permission for analysis'. Analysis or testing of the sample itself could be prohibited and the sample destroyed but any results from the sample that had been used in previous analyses and publications could not be withdrawn.

## *Proxy consent*

As time went on, protocols had to be drawn up to cover obtaining consent from children arriving in clinics with adults other than parents or guardians (such as grandparents) or accompanied by other minors (such as older siblings), and, by 2003, when the children were approaching their teenage years, arriving by themselves. This had implications not only for consent, but also for chaperoning, as the Committee advised that any session involving physical contact (for example anthropometry, which included head, arm, waist and hip circumference measurements) should be chaperoned either by the parent or another member of staff. This was for the protection of both the child and the member of staff conducting the measures. The protocol tried to ensure that the process was as easy as possible for the parents without compromising the consent process. The consent forms and information sheets would be sent in advance to be signed by the parent or guardian, or another form was included giving the person who would be attending with the Study child the authority to sign on their behalf. If the Study child arrived without the relevant forms, there was a process to try to obtain verbal consent on the phone, which was witnessed by a second member of staff. If the parents could not be contacted, the tests were not carried out. There was some concern that staff were unable to be certain of the identity of the person they were talking to on the phone but it was pointed out that checks on identity were not made at the clinics either[15] and no further stipulations were made.

## *Other consents*

As the Study and technology developed, the Committee reviewed and approved other consent processes: photos of Study children could be included on the ALSPAC web site only with parental consent (and without surnames attached)[16] and reminders of clinic visits could be sent by text to mobile phones or by email, again, only with parental consent.[17] The Committee's consideration of the issues involved in obtaining informed consent was hugely time-consuming but surprisingly not because of the policy of broad consent for genetic material, controversial as it was or rapidly became as other studies started conducting similar genetic research. This aspect of consent was accepted within ALSPAC as sensible, pragmatic and ethical. Central to this was the Study participants' trust in the Study investigators; the Committee had an acute awareness of this trust and an unwavering commitment to nurture it in the Cohort. It was the Committee's wish to see all documentation for participants, especially consent forms and accompanying information sheets, that took up so much time as the Study became increasingly complex with substantial numbers of sub-studies built in. As recognised by others (O'Neill, 2003), the appropriate balance between too much and too little information had to be found.

# SEVEN

# Child protection: an observational study?

The principle of non-intervention that was inherent in the design of ALSPAC was soon challenged as child protection and other individual concerns were raised. These concerns arose when Study families were visited at home, attended ALSPAC research clinics or imparted worrying information when answering questions in interviews or questionnaires. The Committee reviewed many cases individually, and from these genuine cases, pragmatic guidelines and protocols evolved.

The design criteria for the European Longitudinal Study of Pregnancy and Childhood (ELSPAC), the consortium to which ALSPAC belonged, stated: 'The Study is observational and should aim to intervene as little as possible in the normal course of the pregnancy and childhood'.[1] Absolute non-intervention was ethically problematic but many of the research questions that were to be asked were specifically included to establish if interventions were appropriate or necessary.

## Family Liaison Team

Some guidelines on intervention were established rapidly in the first few months of ALSPAC's instigation. The ALSPAC 'interviewers', later to be renamed the Family Liaison Team, visited participants' homes to help with the completion of questionnaires and needed some guidance if concerned about participants. Their instructions, almost certainly written by their manager, stated: 'If you come across a situation that worries you, e.g. child abuse, report back to the office. It is not breaking confidentiality'.[2] Presumably, this was not considered to be breaking confidentiality as the information remained within the Study team. These instructions were reviewed by the Committee, who expanded on confidentiality and stated that the interviewer should 'report it to the office but not to anyone else (except of course in the case of an emergency when, for example, an ambulance may be immediately necessary)'.[3] In further discussion, guidelines for Jean Golding (in other words, 'the office') were set out:

> It was decided that certain problems ought to be referred … to Professor Baum or some other medical doctor connected to the study.… the study bore no responsibility to investigate or deal with many of the potential problems … property or drug-related criminal activity, revelations about HIV infection.… Although such matters might cause concern, the importance of maintaining confidentiality was felt to override the desire to intervene. However … there were certain limited situations in which it would be wrong for the study to be held to a policy of non-intervention: for example, if a child were actually abused in the presence of the interviewer. The committee decided that it would not wish to provide a precise list of instances in which Dr Golding should pass on such information: she agreed to discuss sample cases with the group as they arose, in order that the policy might be reviewed. (Committee minutes, September 1990)

Two cases were duly brought to the Committee by Jean Golding in 1995; in both cases, the Committee decided that the policy of non-intervention was appropriate but this was not always to be the case. The first case in May 1995 was described in the minutes:

> An interviewer had expressed concern about a child who demonstrated autistic-type behaviour and whose mother did not

acknowledge that there was any problem. She wondered whether someone ought to be notified especially if early intervention might improve the child's prospects.

Professor Baum was of the opinion that early intervention might not make much difference; he added that the situation was not the same as that involving a life-threatening condition. Mr Hirschmann wondered whether the problem would be likely to be discovered anyway, for example by the child's G.P. It was noted that ALSPAC itself does not have the mechanisms to help. Dr Chambers remarked that to notify the G.P. or health visitor would be to place the difficult burden on them of interfering when their assistance had not been sought. The general view was not to intervene; however, Mrs Bryer asked how the interviewers would react to such a decision. (Committee minutes, May 1995)

The answer to the question put by Mrs Bryer, the first Study mother to join the Committee, is not known, but only a few months later, a very similar concern from another of the interviewers was put to the Committee:

During a home visit to a three-year old child, one of the interviewers formed the impression that the child was developmentally delayed and wondered if the child might have a hearing problem. There was no indication from the mother that she had noticed any problems. In the absence of Professor Baum, Dr Emond was consulted. He thought that early intervention might be of some benefit to such a child and suggested that the health visitor be contacted.

The committee found this case similar to that reported in the minutes of 1 May 1995 and decided that the approach taken then ought to be applied here. ALSPAC's policy in general is not to intervene; mothers should not be asked whether they have noticed problems detected by the interviewer. The Health Service ought to be examining this child in the ordinary course of events and problems would likely be detected at that point (although Mr Hirschmann wondered how many children are actually seen at 3½.) It was also felt by the committee that interviewers needed to be briefed on ALSPAC's policy. (Committee minutes, October 1995)

## Research clinics

The procedure for staff concerned about children evolved and became more formalised with the establishment of the 'Focus at 7' research clinic, where up to 8,300 children were seen over a two-year period. The Committee approved the following statement: 'If a tester has serious concerns about a child's health and safety, he/she will communicate with the clinic manager, the paediatrician in charge or study director in confidence and the issue may then be taken to an appropriate authority and/or the ALSPAC Ethics Committee to decide on action.'[4] By the eight-year clinic, this was expanded further:

If abuse is suspected (sexual abuse or unacceptable physical force used against the child), the child will be told that the information may be passed on to someone who can help him or her. If the information given by the child is ambiguous, the member of staff will attempt to clarify what the child has said. After the session, the member of staff will write down … his or her concerns about the child, without using the child's name or any other identifier.… The report without identifier will be passed to Professor Jean Golding, who will then consult with Dr Alan Emond as appropriate. If they decide to take it further, they will approach … [the] team leader for details which will identify the child. (Committee minutes, June 2000)

Alan Emond was a community paediatrician and close collaborator of ALSPAC, who decided that intervention was necessary on a few occasions and the parents and social workers were contacted. This illustrates, once again, how confidentiality was paramount and participants' identities were protected unless not doing so was considered absolutely necessary.

## Psychologists' sessions

By the 10-year clinic, a formal policy was reviewed and approved by the Committee[5] but this proved inadequate for the types of disturbing problems that the staff were coming across in one particular clinic session. These sessions were conducted by ALSPAC psychologists and included questions on friendships and peer groups, bullying, antisocial activities and depression. Some concerns were presented to the Committee:

- A child being bullied at school, to and from school, including an attempted strangulation, who feels that the school is not doing anything to help them, and scored highly on the depression scale.
- A child disclosing that they do not have any friends, feeling very isolated, and do not feel they can talk to anyone at school when they are attacked and again scoring highly on the depression scale.
- A child with special needs, who presented themselves as rather immature who disclosed that their friends set fire to things and are encouraging them to take part, and that he intends to make a petrol gun and use it. (Committee papers, May 2002)

The staff were restricted to recommending that the child talks to a parent or teacher or phones Childline (a free 24-hour counselling service for children run by the National Society for the Prevention of Cruelty to Children). After considerable discussion and redrafting, the policy was extended and clarified to include a section specifically for the psychology team (see Box 5). This made clear that if the child requested help, their consent was needed for a member of staff to contact their parents before their school or any other body could be approached. If this consent was not obtained and the staff member remained concerned that the child was at risk, the child would be told that someone else would have to be informed and the process of anonymous referral described earlier would be instigated.

---

### Box 5: Section from the ALSPAC Child Protection Policy

**The Psychology Team**

- In the rare cases where the child may want to speak in more detail about their problems. Please say 'I'm sorry I'm not able to help you now. But would you like us to ring somebody at home to talk about this?'
    ◊ If the child does request help it is vital that you find out who they want us to contact at home; mother, father, carer.
    ◊ Then clarify with the child that it would be ok for us to contact the nominated person.
    ◊ At the end of the session check again with the child that it is ok to contact their parents and ask them to let their parents know that someone from Children of the Nineties will phone them.
    ◊ If the child declines this help, explain that we cannot contact the school or anyone else without first informing their parents/carers.
- Skip any potentially upsetting parts of the session.
- If you have concerns that the child may be taking part in behaviours that may risk their health in the future, please pass this information on to the Head of Team, as with any concerns you may have over the child's welfare. (Committee papers, July 2002)

---

The policy was reviewed regularly by the Committee with consideration to different concerns, such as self-harm or suicidal thoughts,[6] psychotic symptoms[7] or general unease by the staff over the level of intervention.[8] ALSPAC's non-interventionist position was observed unless there was evidence that a child was a serious danger to themselves or others.

## Questionnaires

Information that might cause concern from questionnaires was treated differently, although this was not included formally in a child protection policy until 2007. The Committee had decided in 2003 that 'ALSPAC did not have a duty of care should "alarming" answers be given'.[9] The Child Protection Policy of 2007, co-authored by Elizabeth Mumford, stated:

> Data from postal questionnaires and computerised questionnaires completed at the clinics may not be analysed for many years; it takes two years for a complete data set to be collected. Information from these sources, which may in other circumstances cause concern, is never used for any sort of intervention. (Child Protection Policy, July 2007)

Although clearly designed as an observational non-interventionist study, it was established from the very beginning that there were circumstances when intervention was necessary. The Committee were asked to consider the ethical implications of intervention or non-intervention time and time again over the years. During this time, ALSPAC policy formed, although it was not comprehensively documented and formalised as such until after Jean Golding had retired.

# EIGHT

# Disclosure of individual results: foreseen feedback and incidental findings

The Committee's general position of non-disclosure of individual participants' results was soon challenged. On many occasions, they had to review matters concerning the discovery of treatable conditions either foreseen (such as anaemia when analysing blood for haemoglobin levels) or unexpected if something unusual was detected (such as a possible tumour), now known as an 'incidental finding'. After extensive deliberations, their policy was eventually determined: before the disclosure of individual results, data must give clear, unequivocal evidence of an existing or future health problem, *and* the health problem identified must be amenable to treatment of proven benefit. Other cohort studies established since ALSPAC have not always come to the same conclusion.

The discovery of a treatable condition or disease can be ethically problematic for an observational study. This was acknowledged in the very first meeting of the ALSPAC Ethics and Law Committee in April 1990 when it considered:

> Should ALSPAC practice be to always/sometimes/never notify them [participants] (e.g. if a treatable disease is discovered?) ... one view would suggest an obligation to ... inform [the participant] at once, [although] it was possible to argue that

chances were high that any such problem would already have been diagnosed in the ordinary clinical fashion. Problems were more likely to arise in the context of genetic abnormalities, where information gained from the study (and possibly otherwise unavailable to the participants) might be of assistance in deciding whether or not to have any more children. (Committee minutes, April 1990)

Although divulging individual results for a variety of tests was discussed at great length by the Committee on many occasions, genetic abnormalities were never discussed again. The Committee did review an information sheet in 1999 which 'emphasised that no one would be given any results of the genetic tests, whatever they might be. ALSPAC was interested in populations rather than individuals and most of the tests being carried out were in areas that were at present insufficiently understood to provide any meaningful information on an individual level.'[1] So, although the collection and utilisation of genetic data in the context of a population study was a research methodology not used before, the disclosure of individual genetic results took up little of the Committee's time, unlike the many other non-genetic results.

Feedback of individuals' results was also a concern for the Parents Advisory Group that met in May 1990.[2] This parent group did not feel that non-intervention was justified on the grounds of confidentiality in the case of a significant medical problem and wanted assurance that the participant's GP would be notified. The discovery of a 'treatable disease' was a near certainty with some common conditions such as anaemia when testing for haemoglobin levels, while other rare or unexpected conditions were possible but unlikely to be uncovered. An ALSPAC policy concerning the latter, now termed incidental findings, was not considered for some years; initially, the Committee had to decide on how to deal with predictable discoveries.

## Foreseen feedback

Within eight months of their first meeting, the Committee were asked by Jean Golding to decide if disclosure of results was an ethical necessity for an environmental sub-study that intended to measure a variety of indoor air pollutants. These measurements were being made in order to determine the impact on individuals' health. The sub-study was funded by the Department of the Environment, whose usual practice was to disclose all results to participants when undertaking these types of studies. The Committee, when first discussing the sub-study, thought that the results should only be divulged if the pollutant levels were known to be dangerous.[3] The Department of the Environment determined a threshold above which there should be intervention 'although we have no evidence to suggest that the level of the pollutant found in the home is detrimental to health, the level found was unusually high and it would therefore be prudent to investigate the cause and take steps to reduce the concentration of the pollutant e.g. by increasing ventilation.'[4] The ALSPAC Committee approved disclosure above this threshold despite this being contradictory to their initial conclusion that the pollutant level must be known to be dangerous. A similar conclusion was reached when another sub-study on radon was reviewed at around the same time. The National Radiological Protection Board, a non-departmental government body that conducted research and provided information, advice and services around radiological protection, had statutory thresholds for action to be taken. The Committee agreed that parents should be told if their homes had radon levels exceeding this threshold, 'although there was some question about what the "danger level" actually was'.[5]

By 1994, the policy was clarified, as can be seen in a letter from Jean Golding to a collaborator interested in lead levels in children: '… it is totally against the policy of the ALSPAC study to divulge results of any tests to mothers unless there is unequivocal evidence that without intervention, harm will come to the child'.[6] In the UK, there was no screening or legal threshold for intervention, unlike in the US.[7] The Committee discussed what parents should be told about their children's lead levels and decided, '… in keeping with previous decisions of this nature, to inform parents that they would be told if they had very high levels of lead, levels at which present knowledge would clearly indicate the importance of intervention'.[8] The threshold was determined by the collaborator.

Several years later, in yet another sub-study, it was decided that the measurements of electromagnetic fields within homes should be disclosed on request despite the association with ill health being unknown. The collaborator attended the Committee, as documented in the minutes:

[The collaborator] was of the view that participants should be told their electric field measurements if they asked. There was, of course, the further issue of whether this information should be provided even if it was not requested. ([The collaborator] indicated that if his own house had a high rating, he would choose to have it re-wired.) Perhaps study participants should be given this option.

Professor Golding pointed out that it was the usual study policy not to provide results. The significance of various numbers and what their correlation might be to ill health was at present unknown. However, it was decided that there was no sufficiently strong ethical reason not to provide the actual numbers if requested to do so. The engineer might then add that the significance of the numbers was unknown. (Committee minutes, January 1998)

The various decisions to divulge results were not entirely consistent and did not always comply with the ALSPAC policy clearly defined by Jean Golding in 1994 that results should not be divulged unless there was 'unequivocal evidence that without intervention, harm will come to the child'. Although the Committee was finding its way, it seems surprising that, particularly with environmental measures, they were persuaded to ignore their own policy on occasions.

Another early decision to divulge results came after lengthy discussions by the Committee concerning a proposed sub-study that involved an ultrasound scan of the newborn baby's head.[9] The clinical significance of many brain irregularities was unclear but it was decided that 'a list be made of abnormalities which could clearly be diagnosed and particularly of those where early intervention would be to the child's benefit. In such cases, both medical staff and parents should be notified of the existence of the problem.'[10] As the Committee had other concerns about this sub-study (the appropriate time to ask for consent and the response of the parents to the testing), a pilot study was suggested. This was duly conducted and the results reported to the Committee.[11] Eventually, the sub-study was approved, including the limited disclosure of individual results, but the study was not implemented as financial support was not forthcoming. This decision to divulge results was consistent with the yet-undocumented policy as diagnosis and early intervention would be to the child's benefit.

Low haemoglobin indicating anaemia was the first test result that the Committee agreed should be reported to the participant's GP, although it was decided that it was preferable for ALSPAC not to make direct contact with the GP. Participants would be issued with letters to be given to their GPs if they so wished, a practice that was to become commonplace in ALSPAC when individual results were to be divulged. When the Committee was first informed of the sub-study 'Is screening for anaemia in the first two years of life worthwhile?', they rejected any intervention as it was thought that '… it would be more contrary to the spirit of ALSPAC if results were divulged to parents  especially when the precise medical significance of mild, but asymptomatic, anaemia was not known (and was in fact the question being investigated by the study).'[12] A few months later, when the issue of infant anaemia was discussed again, the Committee reversed its decision. It was decided that low haemoglobin results *should* be disclosed if it would warrant further investigation in a clinical situation but also that care must be taken not to give the impression that a clinical service was being offered.[13] This was an important point that was to be emphasised over and over again by the Committee over the coming years: participants should not be given the impression that ALSPAC clinics provided a health check. Jean Golding, in consultation with Alan Emond, Community Paediatrician and ALSPAC collaborator, decided on the haemoglobin threshold warranting disclosure. During these discussions, there was concern that the blood would not be analysed until the end of the sub-study at least 18 months later (although, in fact, analysis of the blood immediately after sampling rapidly became possible). The delay to analyses for a variety of reasons, such as the 'batching' of laboratory tests, and the subsequent implications on the disclosure of results were discussed on occasion but no obvious solution was found.

The infant anaemia sub-study rapidly developed into the 'Children in Focus' sub-study, incorporating a much wider range of measurements. This 10% sample of the cohort children, numbering approximately 1,400, were invited to attend a research clinic, initially at the age of four months and then nine more times in their first five years. Details of the measurements can be found on the ALSPAC website[14] and a summary is given in Figure 2. Each measurement was considered by the Committee before the clinics began, to decide if results should be divulged. Expert collaborators were consulted to determine if there were clinically significant thresholds with effective available treatments. For example, if specific defects were found during the vision tests, immediate referral for treatment by the collaborating ophthalmologist was offered.[15] In the unlikely event of very high plasma cholesterol levels indicating familial hypercholesterolemia being found, referral to the collaborating clinician was suggested[16] but, in this case, the Committee decided not to intervene as treatment at this age was uncharted and such intervention was likely to cause unnecessary stress.[17]

Informing parents of their children's blood pressure results was another early decision by the Committee that would conflict with the Study policy when eventually documented; specifically, results should not be divulged unless there is unequivocal evidence that without intervention, harm will come to the child. The information sheet reviewed by the Committee for the first Children in Focus clinic stated: 'If we find that the blood pressure is unexpectedly high, we will

**Figure 2: Children in Focus clinics: categories of measures (Jean Golding)**

| Category | 4 mths | 8 mths | 12 mths | 18 mths | 25 mths | 31 mths | 37 mths | 43 mths | 49 mths | 61 mths |
|---|---|---|---|---|---|---|---|---|---|---|
| Anthropometry | * | * | * | * | * | * | * | * | * | * |
| Vision | * | * | * | * | * | * | * | * | | * |
| Otitis media with effusion and hearing | | * | * | * | * | * | * | * | * | * |
| Diet | * | * | | * | * | | * | * | | * |
| Cognitive measures | * | | | * | | | | | * | * |
| Blood sample | | * | * | * | | * | | * | | * |
| Day care interview | | | | * | * | * | * | * | * | |
| Dental observation | | | | | | * | | * | | * |
| Skin observation | | | | | | | | | * | * |
| Speech | | | | | * | | | | | |
| Laterality | | | | | | | * | | | |
| Fingerprints | | | | | | | | * | | |
| Skin prick test for allergy | | | | | | | | | | * |
| Lung function | | | | | | | | | | * |
| Fitness | | | | | | | | | | * |
| Parenting measures | | | * | | | | | | | * |

tell you about this so that you can seek appropriate medical advice'.[18] The threshold for such an intervention was established on the advice of an expert, which 'fits in broadly with British Hypertension Society guidelines'[19] and was based on mild hypertension in young adults. Six years later, when plans were being made to invite the whole cohort to the seven-year clinic, the Committee were made aware that there were no reliable norms for this age group and that ALSPAC would be establishing baselines. Nevertheless, the Committee recommended that 'the parent be advised to take their child to the G.P. for re-testing, explaining that there were a variety of reasons for elevated blood pressure, including anxiety'.[20]

Defective hearing, as with anaemia, was a test result that the Committee initially decided should not be revealed at the Children in Focus clinics but was later retracted. This was due to concerns expressed by both parents and clinic staff once the clinic was up and running. The Committee's first discussion when informed of the proposed tests described the dilemma:

> The study planned to look at the problem of otitis media with effusion. It was estimated that 30% of children would be found to be abnormal in the average winter screening. The aim of the study was to discover whether, over time, the treatment or non-treatment of this condition would affect the linguistic ability of the child. There were two complicating factors: first treatment of all those discovered to have the condition would prevent the purpose of the study being fulfilled as there was no control group. However, in addition, there was some doubt about the efficacy of existing treatments. Furthermore, treatment is frequently not carried out until there have been several episodes of otitis media but those screening the children for the study would not know their past history. (Committee minutes, December 1991)

It was important that the treatment on offer was not fully evidence-based and there were questions as to its efficacy; had it been known to be an effective treatment, withholding treatment would almost certainly have been considered unethical.

The matter was left unresolved until further discussion when the Children in Focus clinics were about to begin. The participant information sheets were reviewed and the Committee advised: 'to make very clear … that some results … would not be reported back to the parents [as] some parents might otherwise be misled into thinking that their babies' ears, etc. had been "checked" and found healthy'.[21]

Once the children were attending the clinic and the hearing tests were under way, the staff reported that: 'More and more parents are putting pressure on the staff for hearing test results and are gradually getting more annoyed by the lack of response from us.' [22] Some parents of children who had poor results from the hearing tests had been told by their health visitor that the child's hearing was fine and any behavioural problems were due to something else. In one extreme case, the child was being recommended for a special school. In consultation with the paediatric audiologist who was collaborating with ALSPAC and advising on the hearing tests, it was decided to give parents the results of the hearing tests, including if the child's hearing was within normal limits.[23] By the seven-year clinic (when the frequency of temporary hearing loss due to glue ear is much reduced), the Committee was consulted and only those parents of children showing deficient hearing were given the results.[24] The letters stated that their child's hearing '… was not within normal limits and advisable to have another test done. This will probably be done at school but if you have any concern please ask your G.P., school nurse or health visitor to refer your child to the Child Hearing Centre.'[25]

The confusion around the development of the policy for disclosing individual results was acknowledged by the Committee during the planning of the seven-year clinic when the Committee discussed which results should be revealed to parents:

It was decided that whatever our former policy had been in this area, it was open to us to review and change that policy. The committee chose to maintain the policy of giving test results (if available) to parents where there were 'clear health implications' involved. It was not necessary to limit this to situations where 'efficacious interventions' might be possible. (Committee minutes, March 1998)

At this stage, the Committee again decided that it was not necessary to have 'unequivocal evidence that without intervention, harm will come to the child', as stated by Jean Golding in 1994[26] and eventually incorporated into the documented policy.

## Incidental findings

Incidental findings were discussed by the Committee on a number of occasions. The first, in 1998, was in relation to brain MRI scans proposed to be conducted on a subset of ALSPAC children at the Institute of Child Health in London. The minutes stated that:

It was the policy of the Institute of Child Health to contact parents in any case in which a problem was identified in a scan.... The committee were happy to uphold this policy. However, it was felt important to give parents proper advance notification. They ought to be told ... of the (fairly remote) possibility that something abnormal might be detected and divulged to them. (Committee minutes, September 1998)

A few years later, a senior member of the clinic staff, prompted by a parent's query, asked the Committee for guidelines should anything suspicious be noticed on a DXA scan:

J.G. showed the committee an example of the DXA scan of the skeleton and lungs that a child is given at the Focus at 9 clinic and asked the committee to consider the action that should be taken if something unusual should been seen, for example a tumour. J.H. identified two problems: i) a staff member, and ii) a parent, noticing something out of the ordinary. M.F. presented a further scenario: a parent contacts ALSPAC sometime after the clinic asking why we hadn't noticed a particular abnormality. After some discussion it was decided that the parents should be informed that the clinic staff are not trained to spot abnormalities but if they did notice something odd or if the parents had concerns they should take the scan to their G.P. who would be able to follow it up if necessary. J.G. would draft a letter to the G.P. to be given to the parents in those circumstances. (Committee minutes and draft letter, February 2001)

When a suspected tumour was seen on a DXA scan the following year, Jean Golding immediately showed the scan to the Community Paediatrician, who referred it to a consultant radiographer, who advised further referral to an oncologist.[27] The parent and GP were also informed and when Jean Golding reported her actions to the Committee, they 'commended the procedures and the speed with which they had been implemented'.[28] At about the same time, another incidental finding (a raised white blood cell count, possibly indicating leukaemia) was referred to an expert, who thought that the result much more likely indicated the start of an infection, not leukaemia, and intervention was not advised.[29] This approach of (anonymous) referrals to appropriate experts who then decided if intervention was necessary was eventually incorporated into (informal) policy by Jean Golding.

David Jewell reflected on the Disclosure of Results Policy that was eventually documented, though some time after Michael Furmston and Jean Golding had retired:

"What emerged from this was the need to have a general policy about disclosure of information from research. That policy ... was written by Gordon Stirrat and we have since revised it and it has become very interesting because we have had numerous conversations since with other people involved in different studies where they struggle with the same issue and we worry, at least I worry, because we've taken a minimalist position, that the default which everybody has agreed in ALSPAC is that we should as a general rule not inform people of abnormal findings unless certain specific conditions are met, which is different from a general position which other people adopt, which is in general you *would* inform them." (David Jewell, Oral History Interview, 2012)

ALSPAC was not, in fact, nearly as minimalistic as some other studies, such as UK Biobank (the large national longitudinal study set up in 2006): 'Apart from providing you with the results of some standard measurements made during [your] visit, none of your results will be given to you or your doctors (even if the results do not seem to be normal)'.[30]

The ALSPAC policy that was eventually drawn up[31] was quite clear as to when individual results should be divulged, and included:

- that an item of data gives clear, unequivocal information of an existing or future health problem; and
- that the health problem identified is amenable to treatment of proven benefit.

It took many years, with some contradictory decisions, before the Committee could establish how it should come to consistent decisions on the disclosure of individual results that were not 'contrary to the spirit of ALSPAC'.

# NINE

# Disclosure of individual results: participants' requests

On occasions, the Committee had to review requests for individual results from Study participants, clinicians and lawyers. They thought it prudent to review all such requests as it was for them to decide if, and under what circumstances, information should be disclosed and, in doing so, whether to break the guarantee to keep data anonymous. The risk of the guarantee of anonymity being broken was that this could soon become widely known in such a localised study and the vital trust of the participants in the investigators would be diminished. Despite considerable pressure at times to release results and with conflicting legal opinions, the Committee never felt that an individual's circumstances warranted the disclosure of the information requested.

Over the years, the ALSPAC Ethics and Law Committee were asked to consider many issues relating to the disclosure of individual Study participants' results. Other than the feedback decided in advance or the discovery of an unusual treatable condition, as described in chapter Eight, some participants (or lawyers or clinicians acting on their behalf) requested results to specific tests, such as the disclosure of paternity status.

The disclosure of individual results broke the guarantee of anonymity made to participants as names would necessarily have to be linked to the results (apart from a few results that were obtained in participants' presence and given to them on the spot, such as heights and weights) and the Committee was particularly reluctant to do this unless it was considered absolutely essential. At one time, the University's Information Rights Officer suggested that any participant's requests for individual data should be allowed. This suggestion was not made directly to ALSPAC, but was in answer to a question during a training seminar provided by the University Governance Team.[1] Elizabeth Mumford (an expert on medical law) was consulted and felt that the Information Rights Officer's suggestion was unsound and the Committee chose to ignore it. This is indicative of the tension that built up between the ALSPAC Committee and the higher levels of University Governance, which only became established long after the ALSPAC Committee had been in place.

Individual requests for data were dealt with on a case-by-case basis by the Committee. The first request for release of questionnaire data came from a solicitor representing an unmarried pregnant participant whose partner had died suddenly. She was anxious to ensure that he was declared the father of her unborn child. The partner had completed a questionnaire that included a question on paternity. After considered advice from Elizabeth Mumford (see Box 6), breaking the code was rejected.

**Box 6: Personal reflections (not formal legal opinion) of Elizabeth Mumford regarding release of questionnaire data (Letter to Jean Golding, November 1992, embargoed)**

I see no reason why the solicitor should not formally be told by us that the father filled in an ALSPAC questionnaire. He might also be told that 98.?% of respondents answered the question about paternity in the affirmative. Both of these facts would provide additional supporting evidence. However, I would be reluctant to hand over the actual questionnaire.

### 1) Respecting the man's confidences

There is certainly no reason to divulge the answers to any questions other than that about paternity. There is a 98% certainty that this man gave a positive answer to the paternity question. But if he did not, then I would be extremely unhappy about disclosing that very private admission to anyone, including the mother.

### 2) Preserving the integrity of the study

Once we have disclosed information in these albeit very sympathetic circumstances, then there is no way in which we can rely on the argument that the code is 'unbreakable'. We would have broken our promise to a participant and this would challenge our credibility in agreeing to respect confidences.

### Conclusion

If the court deemed the answer to the paternity question essential to its decision, then it could direct the questionnaire to be produced under subpoena and we would of course be obliged to comply. (It must be added that courts are very reluctant to insist on the disclosure of confidential information in this way.) However, I suspect that the answer to the paternity question will be either (a) unnecessary or (b) inconclusive in any case. Hence, to break our code, just in case it might be of help, would seem unjustifiable.

Some participants occasionally requested access to their own completed questionnaires for a variety of reasons. One mother asked for access in order to provide documentary evidence in a court case in which she was alleging abuse of her child. The minutes stated:

... the Committee recognised that the information was 'hers', however, to offer her access to it was to acknowledge that the study *could* link questionnaires [to participants' names].... the Committee recommended that the mother be sent a blank copy of the relevant questionnaire and be told that a system had been devised in order to make unwarranted access to information impossible; therefore we might not be able to retrieve the information for her.... it was to be pointed out to her that her own questionnaires were unlikely to add any support to her legal case. This it was hoped would dissuade her from further attempts to obtain her responses. (Committee minutes, September 1997)

Another request was made by a clinical psychologist on behalf of a Study mother. The results of her child's psychological tests were requested as the child was possibly suffering from the effects of lead poisoning. The Committee again declined to disclose results (although they said that they would reconsider their decision if there were clinical reasons for releasing the data)[2]:

D.J. was unclear of the assurances that had been given to ALSPAC parents concerning confidentiality and thought that the parents might, although perhaps not in law, be entitled to access data. J.G. explained that although it was technically possible to link data, the parents had been assured that this would not happen. There may be rare circumstances when it would be necessary (if, for example, a blood sample showed the child had leukaemia). M.F. said that it was the task of this committee to decide if circumstances justified breaking confidentiality. He felt that this particular case did not warrant such action as the clinicians on the committee (J.H. & D.J.) felt it was unlikely to make any difference to the clinical management of the child. The committee did have to think in terms of justifying their decision in court although it was unlikely to come to that. M.F. thought a court would be likely to uphold the committee's decision. (Committee minutes, February 2001)

This was one of many occasions when the possibility of having to justify the Committee's decision in court was mentioned. Michael Furmston and Elizabeth Mumford always had the utmost confidence that the Committee's decisions would be upheld.

Further examples of requests for the disclosure of results, also declined, were for serial heights:

J.G. explained to the committee that the request was for two different types of data; i) heights from the self-completion questionnaires (data only fed back under exceptional circumstances and despite previous requests the committee as yet had not approved such action), and ii) Focus@7 measurements which had been fed back at the time. Both types of data would be difficult to retrieve and would involve breaking of ALSPAC's self-imposed rules. M.F. thought the latter was a good reason to refuse the mother's request and suggested J.G. explained that she had been guided by the ethics committee. D.J. thought it was unlikely to make any difference clinically if the exact heights and dates were known but suggested that the mother was told that the committee would review the request again if it came from a doctor. (Committee minutes, July 2001)

Yet another request again indicates how the Committee, although consistently determined to protect the data given to them in confidence, recognised the need to review each request on merit as there may be exceptional circumstances when confidentiality may have to be broken:

K.B. told the committee that a request had been received from a study mother ... whose son is possibly suffering from cerebral palsy. She wanted to know her son's Apgar scores (score which estimates the physical health of a child at birth). ALSPAC has abstracted this information from the medical records. The committee were sympathetic to the mother's request but felt they should not set the precedent of revealing information abstracted from medical records to parents or others. They suggested that J.G. replies to the mother explaining the committee's position and suggesting the child's neurologist writes to the hospital concerned, asking for the Apgar scores and any other relevant information. (Committee minutes, September 2003)

Jean Golding wrote to the Study mother as suggested and included the name of the hospital consultant and hospital contact details.

The ALSPAC Committee's policy on the disclosure of results demonstrates the discord that evolved between the ALSPAC Committee and the University's Ethics of Research Committee (ERC). This Committee was established in 2002, with some uncertainty initially as to the formal relationship between it and the ALSPAC Committee. Eventually, the governance structure was confirmed and the ALSPAC Committee was answerable to the ERC (through another committee – the Faculty Ethics Committee). As Gordon Stirrat recalled:

"They [the ERC] felt that there were things that we were deciding and then giving opinions on that we weren't competent to decide ... and more things should be passed up to them. The area in which we had the biggest dust-up with them was about providing results, individual results.... That caused quite a lot of problems because [the ERC] had lay members on the Committee, who were lawyers, who felt that, in this time of individualism and human rights, these data were owned by the individuals and therefore the individuals should have access to them." (Gordon Stirrat, Oral History Interview, 2013)

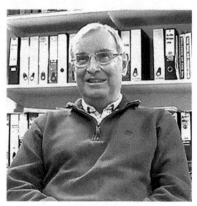

Gordon Stirrat

Despite this conflict of legal opinions and considerable pressure at times to release results, the ALSPAC Committee maintained its position as the preservation of the guarantee of anonymity was considered so crucial to ALSPAC. Nevertheless, the Committee also thought it right to review all such requests and decide if, and under what circumstances, the code should be broken. Frequently, after examining the requests, the Committee came to the conclusion that divulging the information requested would not affect the outcome that the participant was seeking. The Committee never had to justify their decision in court, but both Michael Furmston and Elizabeth Mumford were aware that this was a possibility and would have been prepared to do so.

# TEN

# Participants' problems: people not policies

Individuals' problems that were brought to the Committee's attention vividly illustrated the range of impacts that the Study had on participants but, more significantly, frequently brought up the issue of breaking ALSPAC's guarantee of anonymity. There were some occasions when, for compassionate reasons, the Committee decided that the guarantee should be broken but there were risks in doing so. If it became widely known within the Cohort that the code would be broken on occasions, trust would be jeopardised. The participants' carefully nurtured trust in the research team was critical. Lack of trust was likely to not only increase the attrition rate, but also produce less honest answers in questionnaires, thus jeopardising the scientific value of the Study. As the risks were different in each participant's case, the Committee felt it essential to review each one on a case-by-case basis.

On occasions, the ALSPAC Ethics and Law Committee had to review individual participant issues unrelated to their data or test results, such as requests for help, complaints about the Study processes or concerns by field workers over participants' mental state. The Committee's deliberations over these individual cases made them aware of the range of impacts that the Study had on the lives of individuals, which were not always obvious. It became increasingly important for the

Committee to have this participant perspective and the Study mothers on the Committee were vital in this respect too. Once again, the guarantee made to Study participants in the initial information leaflet that 'no one will be able to link the information that you give us with your name'[1] caused the Committee considerable anguish, particularly concerning some individual requests for help. Although the leaflet had been reviewed and approved by the Committee, Elizabeth Mumford held that this phrase 'came back again and again to haunt us' (Overy et al, 2012, p 75), as stated in Chapter Five.

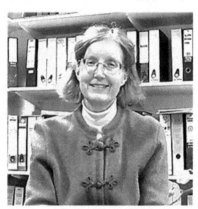

Elizabeth Mumford

## Requests for help

As ALSPAC was designed and conducted as an observational study with minimal interventions, any individual interventions had to be ethically compelling and approved by the Committee before implementation. ALSPAC had a responsibility to participants should they become distressed by aspects of participation in the Study, such as by asking potentially disturbing questions either in questionnaires or at face-to-face interviews, which may require intervention. Practices evolved to deal with such situations, for example, helpline numbers and information about relevant organisations were made easily and discreetly available at clinics or included at the end of postal questionnaires. Volunteers who manned the ALSPAC participant phone 'hotline' were trained to give out similar information. These arrangements were also used when direct requests for help were made that were not necessarily related to distress arising from participation in the Study.

The Committee could be rigid in their denial of help if it involved breaking the guarantee of anonymity. The rationale for this was that in a local population such as ALSPAC, it might become common knowledge that ALSPAC was prepared to break the code for a variety of reasons, including providing help. This might open the floodgates to requests for help but, more importantly, it might jeopardise participants' trust in the researchers.

One request for help to complete questionnaires was made by a 12-year-old sibling of a Study child, whose first language was not English. This was denied as she had made the request on a questionnaire but had signed only her first name.[2] Although stated clearly on the questionnaire that a signature was necessary if a response was required, it seemed harsh to assume that a 12-year-old would understand ALSPAC's requirement for a full signature.

On other occasions, the code was allowed to be broken. One Study mother had given consent for tests to be carried out on her placenta providing that the placenta was eventually returned to her. The Committee decided to allow the code to be broken in order to be able to identify the placenta and return the unused portion. This was despite, as documented in the minutes, 'the concern that other participants, if they discovered that the code could be broken, might fear that the anonymity promised to them might be jeopardised'.[3] On another occasion, a questionnaire was received with a signature on it but no text in the space provided. The participant had not signed any previous questionnaires, indicating that she did not think that a signature was required when completing the questionnaires. Within the questionnaire itself, she had indicated that she had been raped by her father. It was not clear to the Committee if the signature was a mistake or she was asking for help. The Committee decided that she should be contacted asking if she had wanted a response. If this was the case, help could be offered in the usual way, such as supplying appropriate contact numbers to support agencies.[4] To break the code when it was so unclear that help was being requested seemed somewhat inconsistent with the refusal of help for a young girl who had neglected to sign her full name.

Other requests for help were more direct; on one occasion, the Committee reviewed a letter that came to Jean Golding from a child (see Figure 3):

> The committee felt that a letter should be written in reply which assumed that the parents would be likely to read it. The letter should explain that the tests carried out at clinics would not necessarily discover all health problems and that it would be appropriate for the child to be seen by her G.P. J.G. would suggest that the child showed the letter to her parents 'in case they didn't realise how worried she had been'. J.G. would also suggest that the child might be able to talk to someone else about her concerns (another relative, teacher, school nurse) and would include the Child Line telephone number. (Committee minutes, October 2000)

A letter was duly written and reviewed by the Committee, who considered it 'an excellent response'.

**Figure 3: Letter to Jean Golding from a Study Child**

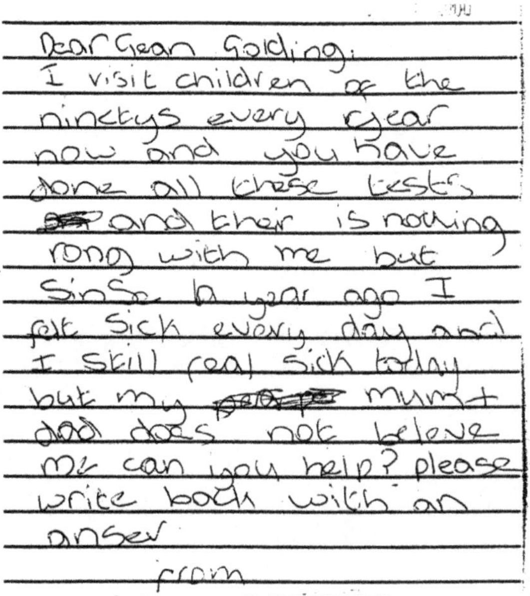
Dear Gean Golding:
I visit children of the
ninetys every year
now and you have
done all these tests
and their is nothing
rong with me but
sinse a year ago I
felt sick every day and
I still real sick today
but my Mum +
dad does not beleve
me can you help? please
write back with an
anser
from

Dear Gean Golding, I visit Children of the ninetys every year now, and you have done all these tests and there is nothing rong with me but since a year ago I felt sick every day and I still feel sick today but my Mum and Dad does not believe me can you help? Please write back with an anser.
from

Another case was referred to Elizabeth Mumford by Jean Golding's Personal Assistant, presumably for legal advice:

> … whilst Jean was away, we had a call from a mother in the study (record of telephone call attached). Whilst this could have waited for JG's return, their plight was featured on the local TV news earlier this week. Jean wondered if you could advise her on what to do. Apparently, this family escaped … [their homeland] a few years ago as political refugees. They are scared to return as the … authorities have videotape showing the parents taking part in demonstrations against the State. The Home Office want them

to go back saying that now there is a change of government it will be safe for them. However the parents argue that they will be detained and interrogated over their participation in these demos (as most of the changes are 'cosmetic' rather than real) and that the children will be taken away and put in orphanages. The mother said she would rather give her children up for adoption in the UK than end up in an orphanage.... They have 28 days to leave the country. The youngest child is 3 and one of the first babies born in the ALSPAC study. As you can see she wonders what effects the 'deportation' may have on him. I guess what she really wants is evidence that the move will have a negative effect on her son to use as ammunition against the Home Office ruling. (Letter to Elizabeth Mumford from Yazmin Iles-Caven, September 1994)

This is one of the more harrowing of participants' stories but, unfortunately, there is no record of the advice given by Elizabeth Mumford or the response from Jean Golding.

## Partner issues

The ALSPAC fathers or partners were not initially enrolled in their own right as they were contacted through the Study mothers. ALSPAC relied on the mothers to pass on the self-completion questionnaires to their partners but ALSPAC was unable to ascertain if this actually happened and were not able to send reminders. Although subsequently regarded as a family study, with many fathers formally enrolled and invited to clinics, during the first years of the Study, some fathers were not fully engaged, as is reflected in the response to questionnaires, which having initially been approximately 10,000, dropped to around 3,650 by the time the children were 11. At this time, 7,500 Study mothers were responding to questionnaires. Some fathers were eager to participate but this could be difficult for partners who had separated from the Study mother and were living apart. It was ethically easier if the break-up was amicable and mothers continued to forward the

'Partners' Questionnaires' and provide information about the child's clinic visits but more difficult if the couple were antagonistic. By 1997, the Committee was asked by Jean Golding to consider couples living apart. Until this time, contact had been through the mother but the Committee was asked to consider if this should change to reflect different family structures. They decided that the mothers should be asked through a newsletter article to supply the names (and presumably contact details) of their partners if separated, although a search through the archived newsletters could find no evidence that this had happened. This is not the only case when a Committee request for an article to be published in a newsletter did not materialise. The minutes record that, 'As to fathers who had written in themselves, it was feared that to accept their offer to participate might run the risk of alienating the mothers if their permission was not sought first'.[5] This proved to be true when, a few months later, the Committee were informed of 'the case of a father whose Study participant wife had left him and who had written in to ALSPAC asking to be sent questionnaires. A subsequent angry letter had been received from the wife, asking "How dare you think of involving him?"'.[6]

At another Committee meeting, it was reported that 'one woman had requested that her husband not be told that the placenta had been taken to be used in the study'.[7] This was not problematic as fathers were not normally informed of the retention of placentas, but it indicates the complexities of family dynamics, not always anticipated.

## Abuse of clinic staff

Abuse of clinic staff was rare but did occasionally occur. An incident involving a Study father becoming abusive to ALSPAC clinic staff was documented by one of the staff involved: 'Man entered office, stopped outside clinic room door. Looked in window. Called out "How much ******* longer? Not hanging about much ******* longer." Tried the door, locked. Shouted out "Don't smile at me. I'll slap your face." Walked out of office towards reception.'[8]

This incident resulted in changes to clinic procedures being drafted by the Clinic Manager:

- To exclude this family from further testing. [Named staff member] to draft a letter for them and circulate it to the rest of the group for comments. [Named collaborator] to be consulted before it is sent.
- Head of Security to be asked whether they or the police should be called for help if needed. (His response was that if the incident is serious enough to need the police anyway, or there is no immediate response from University Security, dial 999. Otherwise phone Security.) The Security number to be placed next to each phone.
- If the receptionist feels threatened by a parent she should quietly leave the reception area; the children are the responsibility of the parent who is with them. She should join the other member(s) of staff and seek help from them (and Security if necessary).
- A meeting of receptionists should be called to discuss the handling of any future such incidents.
- Reception staff to remind parents of the likely length of the test, and to make clear that both parents are welcome to be present. Tester to repeat this welcome to the father/partner.
- No other changes to be made to staffing or to home visits. These were discussed but no decisions made other than to think hard about other studies needing home visits. The general rule was reiterated – that the address to be visited and the estimated return time should be left with a responsible person who would raise the alarm if the tester failed to return.
- Those being required to do home visits need security training before they begin, using the experience, and imagination, of those who have already done them. (Incident Report by Clinic Manager, 1st April 1996)

The document was seen by the Committee, who 'felt it [the document] wholly appropriate'.[9] It was not converted into a formalised policy, but it provided useful clinic guidelines.

## Child's death

Another dilemma that the Committee encountered came after a Study child's death following an asthma attack aged nine. It was suggested to the Committee that it might be scientifically valuable to link the post-mortem results with the mass of longitudinal data that ALSPAC had collected on the child's respiratory health and lung function. If something important was to emerge from such linkage and the results published, it would be extremely difficult to keep the identity of the child anonymous as such deaths are so rare. Linking an individual's results in this way was not the usual ALSPAC policy and the Committee felt that it would weaken ALSPAC's customary position. The chance of discovering a vital 'key' was considered minimal by the respiratory paediatrician who sat on the Committee and the linkage was not approved. Instead, it was suggested that a study looking at the factors associated with severe asthma could be carried out; if all asthmatics needing either intensive care or frequent hospital admissions were selected, then the deceased child's identity could be concealed.[10] This seemed an imaginative proposal for allowing something positive to come out of the tragedy but has not yet been implemented.

## Miscarriage

The Committee had been made aware within their first year of meeting that researchers were interested in both the environmental conditions and psychological aftermath of miscarriage. They had reviewed letters to be sent to mothers who had miscarried,[11] ensuring that they were written with sensitivity. Six months later, other researchers had proposed investigating electromagnetic forces possibly associated with miscarriage. Jean Golding informed the Committee that 95% of those who had suffered miscarriage were prepared to continue in the

Study.[12] The Committee were then asked to consider an individual case: a participant had miscarried and her mother had contacted ALSPAC requesting no further contact. The Committee discussed if the daughter should be 'asked her views on the matter'. It was decided that it would be best to contact the participant's health visitor before contact was made.[13] It is not known if this particular participant was contacted, but it illustrates the importance that the Committee gave to each individual participant's involvement in the Study.

## Guarantee of anonymity

Some of the individual issues that were brought to the Committee's attention were straightforward requests for help that did not compromise the guarantee of anonymity, such as the child's letter to Jean Golding or abusive behaviour in the clinic. Other requests, though, again brought up the issue of breaking the code and, with it, the Committee's self-imposed rules. Michael Furmston believed 'that it was the task of this committee to decide if circumstances justified breaking confidentiality'[14] and Jean Golding therefore brought to the Committee any case that required this decision. There were some discrepancies in the Committee's decisions, sometimes agreeing to break the guarantee of anonymity, albeit for compassionate reasons, and sometimes strictly sticking to the guarantee, however harsh. Consistency in this decision-making could perhaps have been achieved if there had been a more formal risk assessment should the guarantee of anonymity be broken. The fear was that if it became widely known within the Cohort that the code could be broken and under some circumstances would be, trust would be jeopardised. This was likely to both increase the attrition rate and produce less honest answers in the self-completion questionnaires. The risks of these outcomes were different in each participant's case and a consistent assessment of risk with guidelines as to when the code should be broken might have prevented the Committee, as Elizabeth Mumford described, being haunted by the guarantee of anonymity.

# ELEVEN

# External databases: anonymous linkage

Linkage to external or third-party databases was an important aspect of ALSPAC's methodology, but although consent on an opt-out basis was acceptable when ALSPAC began, this became inadequate over time as the ethical issues involved in medical research became more prominent and processes for more comprehensive protection of patients developed. This was exemplified by the creation by the Government of the Patients Information Advisory Group (PIAG), which could decide if National Health Service (NHS) records could be accessed by researchers without patients' specific opt-in consent. Informed opt-in consent from ALSPAC participants for linkage to health, education and other third-party databases, as established now within ALSPAC, would perhaps have gone a long way to alleviating the ethical issues that challenged the Committee on a number of occasions.

Some ALSPAC statisticians linked ALSPAC data to publicly available databases, such as Indices of Multiple Deprivation (the deprivation level of the neighbourhood) or the proximity of power lines to homes. These linkages did not pose ethical problems as they did not require consent from the participants and were publicly available. Linkage to other third-party data was less straightforward and did require consideration by the Committee.

## Health records

From the very beginning, health data were made available to ALSPAC from local NHS databases. Linkage to the 'Child Health' database (used extensively by Health Visitors) was integral to the methodology of ALSPAC and ethical approval was not considered necessary. As has been described previously, scrutiny by ethics committees was somewhat relaxed in 1990. The database was checked weekly and used to identify stillbirths and perinatal and infant deaths, thus preventing any inappropriate communications with recently bereaved mothers. Enrolled mothers who had delivered safely were sent congratulatory cards.

The database used by midwives was validated by ALSPAC against the paper records and proved to be both inaccurate and inadequate for ALSPAC purposes, so the paper records were used for abstracting obstetric data. Obtaining information from medical records was mentioned in two of the three initial applications to the Local Research Ethics Committees (LRECs): 'Objective measures of child health (e.g. medical history) and development (e.g. HV [Health Visitor] screening) will be used wherever possible or appropriate. Data on specific medical problems will be ascertained from medical records'. On one of these two forms, an additional handwritten clause followed the typed text: 'after parental consent has been obtained'.[1] The consent obtained was 'opt-out', which was quite accepted by the LRECs at the time; previously, much epidemiological research using health records gained no consent at all and participants were not aware that their records were being viewed. The wording giving ALSPAC participants the option to opt out was far from clear. The initial leaflet to participants concerning enrolment, which was reviewed and amended by the ALSPAC Committee, contained brief information concerning linkage to hospital and other health records:

> We will know how your pregnancy progresses from the hospital records, and details of your baby and how he or she develops from the child health records. These will not give us enough

information on you and your baby though, and we will be sending you questionnaires asking for details. (Initial Participant Information Booklet)

On the following page, there was an option to opt out, although it was not clear that this applied to health records: 'Unless you tell us that you definitely don't want to take part, we will be sending you a questionnaire in a few days time. Other questionnaires will follow in the next few months'. This information giving Study mothers the option to opt out has been exaggerated by some over the years. The published 'Cohort Profile' of the ALSPAC mothers (Fraser et al, 2012) states: 'The information sheets given to the women in pregnancy stated that data from medical records would be abstracted, unless she specifically indicated that she did not want this to occur'.

In 1992, the Committee were reminded of the opt-out consent when they considered (and rejected) accessing the medical records of women who had miscarried prior to joining the Study:

Some of the progress of study participants will be tracked through a study of their hospital records. Participants are told in the initial brochure that researchers will use such records as a source of information; thus it is presumed that if they agree to participate, they have consented to what would otherwise be a breach of confidence on the part of the hospital.

The question presently arising is whether ALSPAC may have access to the records of those women who miscarried prior to joining the study, particularly in order to examine the sort of help such women are given. It would seem insensitive to approach them at that time to ask explicit consent. However, the Committee was of the view that, as these women had done nothing to imply consent, to ask for their records would mean that the study was inducing a breach of confidence. (Committee minutes, July 1992)

The Committee, including the two lawyers, seemed clear that a possible breach of confidence when accessing records would be on the part of the hospital, not ALSPAC, even if 'induced' by ALSPAC. As time went on, there was widespread and increasing concern nationally about consent (or lack of it) to access medical records for research purposes, which culminated in the formation of the PIAG by the Department of Health in 2001. This powerful Committee could authorise the common law duty of confidentiality to be set aside in specific circumstances for research purposes, specifically allowing NHS records to be accessed by researchers without patients' consent. During its existence, PIAG created considerable difficulties for public health researchers and epidemiologists, for example, it took 18 months to obtain a decision from PIAG for one major research project within the same University department as ALSPAC (Department of Social Medicine). As stated by a departmental colleague when a description of this process was published in the *Journal for Medical Ethics* (Metcalfe et al, 2008): 'Such delays pose near insurmountable difficulties to grant funded research, and in our case £560 000 of public and charitable money was spent on research staff while a large part of their work was prohibited until the third year of a three year grant.'

ALSPAC continued to collect data from medical records on the initial opt-out consent, without objection from the local maternity hospitals and without exemption from PIAG.

The team of ALSPAC staff, mostly nurses and/or midwives, who abstracted data from medical records was fully aware of the wording in the initial information leaflet. They were concerned that the information was somewhat misleading and that many ALSPAC mothers would not realise that their medical records were being, or had been, accessed by ALSPAC. The team felt strongly that it was unacceptable to access records if the women had withdrawn from the Study during pregnancy but not if they had withdrawn at a later date as, by this time, it was quite possible that their data could already have been abstracted. Surprisingly, even to the author, who was supervising this team at the time, this matter was not referred to the Ethics Committee. The data abstractors came to their own conclusion regarding the ethics of their work and did not collect data from the medical records of those mothers who had refused in pregnancy.

In 1993, the Ethics Committee was asked to advise on another matter relating to medical records, which tied in with their deliberations concerning identifying mothers through their questionnaire data:

> The committee was asked whether it would be acceptable to check doctor's notes (e.g. about early bleeding in pregnancy) and to compare these with the mothers' responses in the questionnaires. This was felt to be acceptable, as it involved putting information into the computer rather than taking it out. (Committee minutes, August 1993)

It is unclear from the minutes exactly what process was approved by the Committee but it is assumed that the linkage was carried out anonymously in accordance with the usual principles of the Ethical Divide, as described in Chapter Five.

## Office for National Statistics

The Office for National Statistics (ONS), a non-ministerial government department, provided information to ALSPAC concerning mothers who developed cancer or who had died. ALSPAC had supplied a list of participating mothers to the ONS without referral to the Committee. This release of ALSPAC participants' identities only became an issue later regarding linkage to education data. Consent from participants to access the data was not necessary until 2005, when the ONS asked ALSPAC to endeavour to obtain consent from the Study mothers. If participants did not reply, the ONS would supply ALSPAC with data under 'Section 60 Support'. This was an exemption clause in the Health and Social Care Act allowing NHS data to be used without signed consent. The consent form was carefully worded to cover consent for both Study mothers and Study children 'to follow up my health status and keep in touch with my child/children and me'. This form was approved by the Committee, who were impressed with the breadth of the consent.[2] The Committee encouraged broad consent, feeling that it was best not to overload participants with frequent requests if it could be avoided.

## Education records

It appears that the Committee's awareness of ALSPAC's access to educational data, specifically school entry and Standard Assessment Tests (SAT) results from the National Pupil Database, happened quite arbitrarily. They knew ALSPAC collected data through schools as they had reviewed questionnaires sent to teachers and head teachers concerning various aspects of the school environment and ethos, as well as data on individual children.[3] They only became aware of the other educational data sources when the Committee was asked to advise on the age that a child could give consent for linkage to educational records. Parents had been asked at the Focus at 7 clinic to consent to ALSPAC linking their child's education records to ALSPAC data and one parent had refused to consent to linkage after the child reached 10 years old unless their child had given consent themselves. The lawyers on the Committee advised that the law was unclear on this matter. It was also observed that the Data Protection Act 1998 was 'confusing, particularly concerning epidemiology and public health'. Although 'there was a general agreement within the committee that it would be better to involve the children soon rather than leave it until they were older',[4] there does not seem to have been any further action on gaining consent from the children themselves. The Committee rather vaguely recommended that the children should be consulted at the Focus at 10 clinic some years away.

The following year, the Committee again discussed consent for linkage to educational records. Jean Golding explained that over 3,000 Study families had not attended the Focus at 7 clinic and consent had therefore not been obtained. She suggested writing to these 3,000 families to inform them that the educational data would be used unless they objected (opt-out consent). Most of the Committee felt that this was not adequate and it was suggested that the participants should be written to in the first instance asking for signed consent. If they did not reply, they should be contacted by phone. The Chair asked that the Committee review the process again after these steps had been taken, by which time, the numbers involved, he presumed, would be considerably reduced.[5] This advice was not acted upon immediately and after a further nine months, another issue concerning these data emerged. This time, it was the ALSPAC statisticians who felt that the wording of the consent form was vague and they were uncertain how they could use these data.

This exemplifies the way in which ALSPAC operated at its best: staff anxieties about ethical issues were taken seriously and the issues were brought to the attention of the Committee. In this instance, it meant that the consent form was viewed by the Committee, who, surprised that it had been approved, asked to see the minutes of the meeting that had dealt with the consent form and any supporting papers.[6] These did not materialise as the Committee had not been asked to review the form. At the time the Focus at 7 clinic was set up, ethical review of such paperwork had regrettably not become embedded in the ALSPAC clinic procedures. The consent form was confusing and would almost certainly have been amended had the Committee seen it before it was put into use. Not only did it serve a dual purpose – (1) consent for linkage to educational records and (2) consent for linkage to medical records – but it also contained a phrase unlikely to have been approved by the Committee: 'This permission will remain valid until my child becomes 16'. Some Committee members thought that the wording of the form implied that consent was being asked for any medical record that the school held (see Box 7).

---

**Box 7: Focus at 7 consent for health and educational records presented to the Committee in March 2003**

Consent

*FOCUS AT 7*

I understand that the Children of the 90s study may be contacting

a) my child's school, and

b) may look at his/her medical records.

(delete if either not applicable)

I understand that any information will be kept in the strictest confidence, and will be used only for producing statistical information. This permission will remain valid until my child becomes 16.

If I should change my mind at any point I will be free to do so.

Signed...................................................... Date ......................

Your name in full ...........................................................

I.D. ................................................................................

Relationship to child ......................................

---

Once again, the Committee recommended written consent to be obtained using a new form that kept consent for educational and medical linkage quite separate. Although Jean Golding said that she would concentrate on the education consent and would draft a new form and circulate it to Committee members before the next meeting, this did not happen. Instead, Professor Dieter Wolke, ALSPAC Head of Psychology, attended a subsequent Committee meeting describing how scientifically important it was to link these educational data with other ALSPAC data. Jean Golding then described the difficulty and expense involved in gaining written consent from all parents and, as ALSPAC anonymised all data before links were made, written consent was not required under the Data Protection Act. Eventually, the Committee were persuaded, mostly on pragmatic grounds (in this instance, the expense involved) to inform participants of ALSPAC's intention to link to educational records through the regular ALSPAC newsletter with a clear option to opt out.[7] On this occasion, the Committee did take financial considerations into account, although it is questionable as to whether this should influence their decisions. Michael Furmston had been known to say that it should not, yet if important scientific research was impossible to undertake due to stringent Committee rulings when alternative ethical strategies could be implemented, this could also be considered unethical. The Committee reviewed articles for both the participants' newsletter and the newsletter for professionals, which was sent regularly to local health and educational professionals, as well as ALSPAC collaborators.[8] The latter was published but it seems that the article for the participants' newsletter was not, although it is not clear why. It is highly likely that this was an oversight rather than a deliberate refusal to comply with the Committee's advice, but it does suggest that follow-up of the Committee's advice could or should have been more effective.

In 2003–04, there was a confusing episode concerning access to educational data. It is unclear if this was an example of i) inconsistency in the Committee's decision-making or ii) their determination to protect ALSPAC participants. One of ALSPAC's collaborator's projects involved identifying if and when developmental impairments in the Cohort children had been suspected and diagnosed. This included identifying ALSPAC children with special educational needs through Bristol City Council (BCC). The Council were unwilling to release information unless it was confirmed that the child was part of the ALSPAC cohort and a 'Fair Processing Letter' sent. This letter gave the participants an opportunity to opt out of the research and not allow educational details to be passed on to ALSPAC. The Committee would not allow ALSPAC to give a list of ALSPAC participants to the BCC as this was considered confidential information: 'Michael Furmston felt that the issue of trust, whether in the BCC or another institution was irrelevant; the ALSPAC participants had given information on the understanding that it was confidential and therefore their names and addresses should not be revealed.'[9] The Committee were reminded by Jean Golding that a list of participants had been sent to another external organisation, the ONS, with the Committee's permission in order that ALSPAC could be informed of cases of cancer and deaths. If the Committee had sanctioned the release of participants' identifiers to the ONS, it would have been quite inconsistent not to allow the release of similar information to the BCC. There is no evidence in the Committee minutes that they had ever been asked about the release of identifiers to the ONS and so it is more likely that they were taking a principled position on the guarantees of confidentiality that had been made to the Cohort. The impasse with the BCC was resolved by liaison with the Department for Education and Skills (DfES), who had most of the information required by the collaborator. The lists were matched through an independent third party (the Fischer Trust) that the DfES used under similar circumstances. This solution had been suggested to the BCC but they had rejected the suggestion. This was another pragmatic solution by the Committee that went some way to meeting their concerns, although the list of ALSPAC participants did have to be released to a third party (the Fischer Trust), which they had initially categorically ruled out.

Linkage to external or third-party databases was an important aspect of ALSPAC's methodology, as noted in the initial ethical application forms to the LRECs and information booklet for Study mothers. Consent on an opt-out basis for linkage to health data was acceptable at that time but this gradually came to be considered inadequate. The Committee, as always, dealt with ethical issues as they emerged during the running of the Study but there was inconsistency in their decision-making. Although the release of the list of ALSPAC participants' identities to the ONS was not sanctioned by the Committee, when they were made aware of it, they seemed unconcerned. When a similar process was required, albeit to a local, not national, organisation (the BCC), much concern was expressed. The compromise eventually agreed upon used an independent third party to match lists, which inevitably involved the release of the identities of the ALSPAC Cohort anyway. With hindsight, informed consent from participants for comprehensive linkage to health, education or other third-party databases would have gone a long way to alleviating the ethical issues confronting the Committee and eliciting such inconsistencies.

# Part Three
# Beyond policy:
# a broad remit

# TWELVE

# Retention of the Cohort: incentives or inducements

Keeping attrition rates low was crucial to the scientific value of ALSPAC and has contributed to its outstanding success and international recognition. The Committee supported ALSPAC staff in their constant endeavour to this end by keeping the Study participants informed, engaged and enthusiastic. This was achieved by cultivating media coverage, including publicising scientific papers, issuing regular participant newsletters, creating the Discovery Club for the Study children and, where necessary, sensitive contact with individual Study participants. Reimbursements for time and inconvenience were given, as were small rewards for participation in the Study. When the rewards were assessed, the fine line between incentives and inducements had to be negotiated. The Committee considered that inappropriate rewards could make the cohort devalue the Study rather than increase their appreciation of it. They believed that altruism should always be emphasised as this was a powerful motivator for Study participants.

As with all cohort studies, keeping attrition rates low is crucial to the scientific merit of ALSPAC as it maximises statistical power and minimises bias. Although not stated explicitly, this was considered an ethical matter, certainly by Jean Golding. Should participants withdraw from the Study, data already contributed by all Study participants would be devalued. Fewer participants would reduce the power of the statistical analyses as the vital longitudinal nature of these data would be limited. Keeping attrition rates low creates particular challenges in longitudinal studies as cohort participants are frequently studied for decades or throughout their whole lives. Members of the ALSPAC Ethics and Law Committee were acutely aware of this fundamental issue and it influenced almost every aspect of their work. Broad concepts were endorsed, such as the importance of establishing participants' trust in the researchers, protecting them from being overly burdened and ensuring that all written information was easy to read for both children and adults with a wide range of abilities and education. That said, the regular newsletters that were sent to the participants and considered vital to the retention of the Cohort were not reviewed by the Committee before publication. Of course, members of the Committee who were Study mothers did see the parents' newsletters, but on no occasion did they bring to the Committee's attention any concerns.

Local and national media coverage, as well as more direct feedback of published results, was considered equally important in keeping the Cohort engaged and enthusiastic. The Committee rarely influenced the media coverage but were aware that adverse publicity or breaches in confidentiality in such a localised population could have disastrous effects on Cohort retention rates. This led to great care and consideration when their attention was brought to individual participants' requests or problems, as described in Chapter Ten. All these strategies were recognised as an effective method of reducing attrition rates by encouraging participants' identification with the Study and their understanding of the importance of their contributions.

ALSPAC employed a team of staff (the Family Liaison Team), initially to ensure enrolment rates were high and then specifically to keep attrition rates low. The Committee were aware of most aspects of their work, including prioritising the more vulnerable participants and thus keeping involved those who might easily have abandoned the Study due to temporary or permanent stresses (such as illiteracy, mental or physical illness, bereavement, multiple births, large families, or poverty). Ethical issues that arose from this aspect of the Team's work have mostly been described elsewhere, in particular, the child protection issues described in Chapter Seven. The Public Relations Team worked alongside the Family Liaison Team and was equally dedicated to keeping attrition rates low. This team was responsible not only for publicity and media liaison, but also for the newsletters. Both teams were acutely aware of attrition rates, as were the more senior staff involved with the annual Focus Clinics.

## Incentives

Out of the determination to keep the Cohort participants involved and enthusiastic, in recognition of their time and effort dedicated to the Study and to make them feel valued and appreciated, small gifts were offered after attendance at the clinics. These would be inexpensive toys such as 'stretchy men' for the children or pens with the Children of the 90s logo for the adults. Although not documented anywhere, it seems that it was understood that gifts should not be disproportionate: if obtaining the gift was the reason for participating in that aspect of the Study, it was likely that the gift had been misjudged and could be considered unethical. There are subtle distinctions between reimbursements, incentives and inducements that the Committee had to tackle more frequently, both as the Cohort children got older and as the nature of the data collections became more complex. Reimbursements for travel may seem straightforward but, for example, when taxis from participants' homes to the clinic (which could be 20–30 miles away) or train fares and overnight hotel accommodation in London were on offer, could these be judged as inducements? In both these cases, these reimbursements were judged to be ethical and not regarded as inducements, and were approved by the Committee.

The Committee was not usually involved in deciding what these gifts should be; it was assumed that the staff who made these decisions would discern what was appropriate, in that the gifts were not disproportionate or coercive, but specific incentives were occasionally brought to the Committee's attention. On one occasion, the Committee was asked to consider the reward for a sub-study that involved 200 children wearing activity monitors for one week during each season of the year. The Committee was asked if it would be acceptable to give the participants a token for a 'Four Seasons Pizza'; a popular pizza at the time with toppings representative of each season on each quarter of the pizza. Due to the increasing concern by health professionals and others about the levels of obesity in the population, the Committee understandably felt that tokens for pizzas would give the wrong message; tokens for activities (swimming, skating, bowling) were discussed but it was thought that these rewards might influence the results. Eventually, the collaborator was asked to use 'neutral' rewards, for example, CDs or cinema tickets.[1]

More problematic for the Committee was the disclosure of clinical results. Although clinical results were generally not disclosed except under the strictest of criteria (see Chapters Eight and Nine), on-the-spot results of certain clinical measures, such as heights and weights, were disclosed to participants. In fact, the children attending the Focus Clinics were provided with booklets in which to document specific measures (see Figures 4 and 5). Clinic staff reported these booklets to be popular and as enhancing the clinic experience for the children. Positive experience in the clinics not only encouraged the children to attend future clinics, but, if they discussed their experience with their peer group, many of whom would also be Cohort members, could also positively affect clinic attendance rates. There is some evidence that one clinic, which was not much enjoyed by participants, had considerably lower attendance rates due to this informal information exchange. The seven-year clinic was attended by 8,297 children. This dropped to 7,487 at the eight-year clinic and recovered to 7,725 at the nine-year clinic. The clinic for eight year olds involved much time spent on measuring intellectual abilities (IQ, attention, executive function, speech and language) and ascertaining behaviour, attitudes and non-verbal skills (friendships, bullying, anti-social activities, gender behaviour, self-image, non-verbal accuracy), leaving little time for physical measures. The only physical measure was a bronchial challenge, which involved inhaling methacholine, inducing a reduction in lung function that was not considered pleasant. The Committee, alongside others planning the subsequent clinics, tried to ensure that there was a good balance between physical and psychological measures; this was not always easy as it was ALSPAC collaborators' interests and financial contributions that largely dictated the measures to be implemented at the clinics.

### Figure 4: Example page from Focus at 7 booklet

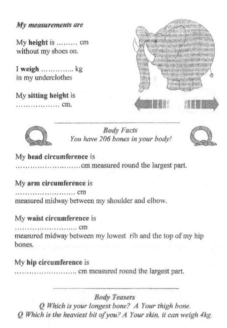

*My measurements are*

My **height** is ......... cm
without my shoes on.

I **weigh** .............. kg
in my underclothes

My **sitting height** is
.................. cm.

*Body Facts*
*You have 206 bones in your body!*

My **head circumference** is
..........................cm measured round the largest part.

My **arm circumference** is
......................... cm
measured midway between my shoulder and elbow.

My **waist circumference** is
......................... cm
measured midway between my lowest rib and the top of my hip bones.

My **hip circumference** is
......................... cm measured round the largest part.

*Body Teasers*
*Q Which is your longest bone?  A Your thigh bone.*
*Q Which is the heaviest bit of you? A Your skin, it can weigh 4kg.*

**Figure 5: Example page from Focus at 7 booklet**

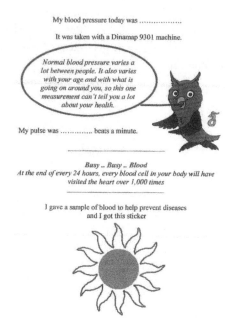

My blood pressure today was .................

It was taken with a Dinamap 9301 machine.

*Normal blood pressure varies a lot between people. It also varies with your age and with what is going on around you, so this one measurement can't tell you a lot about your health.*

My pulse was ............. beats a minute.

*Busy .. Busy .. Blood*
*At the end of every 24 hours, every blood cell in your body will have visited the heart over 1,000 times*

I gave a sample of blood to help prevent diseases and I got this sticker

## The Discovery Club

Another highly successful and popular method of keeping the Study children engaged with the Study and therefore attrition rates low was the 'Discovery Club', which was instigated in 2000 when the children were eight to nine years old. Once enrolled in the Club (by returning a form included in the newsletter or at a later date online), the children would receive a membership card, badge, folder, newsletters and the opportunity to enter many competitions. They were also entered into a monthly prize draw for returning questionnaires. The Committee were told about the Club and shown the form, which made it quite clear that there would be a prize draw, but, surprisingly perhaps considering their major objections a few years later, no objections were made. The Committee's only concern was that it might attract more girls than boys.[2] This proved to be the case, with approximately 500 more girls enrolling in the Club (53% girls and 47% boys). The Club encouraged much active participation by the children, such as: sending in photos and news; taking part in swimming galas, charity bike rides or football tournaments; playing online games; and entering competitions. There was substantial emphasis on the latter and, at one time, a monthly competition was instigated for such things as the funniest joke or best name for the laboratory's DNA robots. There were impressive prizes available, including a helicopter ride, a week-long course at the local science centre culminating in making a film and tickets for various music and other events. The ALSPAC staff ensured substantial media coverage and cultivated good working relationships with the local media, such as arranging for the children's weather pictures to appear on the local television news.

The Discovery Club continued beyond Jean Golding's retirement but in the six years up until then, it rarely came to the Committee's attention. Once, Jean Golding presented a 'fact finder' booklet that she thought could be sent via the Discovery Club and used as an *aide memoire* to help the children fill out their questionnaires; it was not intended to be returned. The Committee had many criticisms (too dry, too culturally specific) and although Jean Golding said that she would redraft it, it was abandoned. On another occasion, when the Committee were discussing the problematic issue of gaining informed consent for immortalised cell lines, it was 'agreed that the Discovery Club should be used to inform the children about DNA and the many issues involved; confidentiality should be re-emphasised'.[3] This would have reached most children still actively participating in ALSPAC, with over 8,000 enrolled in the Discovery Club.

The Discovery Club was brought to the attention of the Committee one further time concerning bicycle helmets. The Club had advertised 'Bristol Biggest Bike Ride', a non-competitive cycling event that 300 Study families had said they would like to join representing Children of the 90s. The team organising this had negotiated a discount on cycle helmets from a firm approved by both the Royal College of Paediatrics & Child Health and the Royal College of Surgeons and wanted to offer them to the Study families at the discounted price. The Committee approved this after checking that ALSPAC would not be liable if a child was injured but also noting that there was some evidence that helmets did not make cycling safer. T-shirts with the Children of the 90s logo were issued to the families and the event was covered by the local media – another example of highly successful promotion of the Study through the Discovery Club by the Public Relations Team.[4]

## The prize draw

As the children became older and their lives busier, response rates to questionnaires and clinic attendance levels understandably dropped, with concern by some staff that this would be exacerbated by the frequency of postal questionnaires that it was necessary to send at times. As with the clinics, much of the information collected by questionnaires was dictated and funded by collaborators. In 2005, the Committee reviewed a request from the Public Relations Team to consider a prize draw for children completing questionnaires. This was towards the end of Jean Golding's and Michael Furmston's era and the Publicity Team consisted of relatively new staff members. Perhaps unknown to them and certainly forgotten by any others who might have known (Jean Golding, the author and the Study mothers on the Committee), a monthly prize draw of £25 had been implemented in October 1997 for participants returning questionnaires. This had not been referred to the Committee. The winners' names were published in the newsletter and this incentive was still being implemented in May 1999, although it is uncertain as to how long it continued. When consulted in 2005, the Committee were unambiguously against implementing a prize draw and even less enthusiastic when asked to consider 'Fundraiser Discount Books' (books of tokens) a few months later, as can be seen in the minutes:

> The committee reviewed the draft invitation to enter a prize draw. This had been suggested by the ALSPAC publicity team, as they thought it might improve the response rate from study children who were about to receive several questionnaires in

quick succession. H.B. thought this was unlikely to increase the response rate and most of the committee felt it might have negative repercussions as the cohort were used to being informed that their participation was an important contribution to science. (Committee minutes, May 2005)

The committee reviewed the Discount Books, a suggested alternative to book tokens that are given to study participants at the clinics currently. Several members were concerned about the time limits on the vouchers, as from their own experience, they did not feel good if they did not use vouchers within the deadlines. Many of the committee members were not happy about the general impression of the books and felt that, as with the prize draw discussed recently, altruism should be emphasised. Some of the committee thought that the nature of these rewards is vital; the wrong sort of rewards can make the cohort devalue the study rather than increase their appreciation of it. The committee felt that book and CD tokens are more appropriate gifts. (Committee minutes, July 2005)

The ALSPAC prize draw illustrates the Committee's ineffectiveness at times as they relied on Jean Golding to bring issues to their attention and if this did not take place, as with the early implementation of a prize draw, important consideration of the ethical implications was not only bypassed, but also not assimilated into the ethos of ALSPAC staff.

The Committee supported ALSPAC staff in their constant endeavour to keep attrition rates low by keeping the Study participants engaged and enthusiastic. The Family Liaison and Public Relations Teams used a variety of methods to achieve this, such as newsletters, the Discovery Club, publicising scientific papers and other media coverage, not all of which were reviewed by the Committee. Incentives were sometimes reviewed by the Committee to ensure that they were proportionate and appropriate but these judgements were mostly made by ALSPAC staff. The emphasis on altruism was always considered an equally important aspect of retaining the Cohort as any of the other methods employed.

# THIRTEEN

## Commercial collaborations: selling our souls

Collaboration with commercial companies, as long as there were strict rules about publication without veto, was standard practice within universities when ALSPAC was founded and not considered controversial by Jean Golding or her many advisory committees. There were few objections from the Study participants, who were made aware through the newsletters of these collaborations, as well as donations, both financial or in kind, from mostly local companies. Throughout the 1990s, there was increasing pressure from the large research funders, such as the Medical Research Council (MRC), to provide 'open access' to data and thus increase collaboration with commercial companies. This did concern the Committee as it raised the possibility of ALSPAC not only losing control of data, but also breaking guarantees given to the participants. After the Committee met with representatives of the MRC and explained the ethical issues involved, no changes were required and collaborating with commercial companies continued as before.

Jean Golding and the ALSPAC Steering Committee always regarded collaboration with commercial companies as acceptable if the companies did not influence any publications coming out of the sponsored research. This position was not due to the lack of core funding that ALSPAC had to endure in the early days as, long before ALSPAC was set up, Jean Golding accepted financial support from commercial companies on this principled basis. Even during the final planning and piloting stage of ALSPAC, she had to be firm with one large international pharmaceutical company who disputed her results when they showed that the company's product was associated with childhood cancer (Golding et al, 1992). Commercial collaborations continued with ALSPAC from its beginning, mostly harmoniously, without being specifically brought to the attention of the Study participants or Ethics and Law Committee. Funding for research on this basis was well established within universities and Jean Golding did not regard it as controversial.

Endorsements by commercial companies came to the attention of the Committee in 1995 when a small supermarket chain expressed interest in subsidising the cost of producing the ALSPAC newsletter. Jean Golding informed the Committee that 'sponsors had supported the study for some time, but the issue of having a sponsor's name included on something that was sent to the parents might ... appear to compromise the independence or integrity of the study'. None on the Committee had any particular objection to this particular supermarket but 'Professor Baum said that he would strongly oppose the use of certain sponsors, such as producers of baby milk formula.... It was generally felt that, if possible, it would be better to include the name of several sponsors rather than just one.'[1] At the time, there was a prominent campaign to boycott one multinational producer of formula milk (Nestlé) as they were seen to be responsible for causing infant illness and death in poor communities, particularly in the developing world, by promoting bottle feeding and discouraging breastfeeding. This boycott continues today. In the previous year, Jean Golding had included in the regular newsletter that was sent to Study participants a brief item on ALSPAC's relationship with commercial companies. It was included in a section entitled 'Your comments':

> One mother felt that if answers are being given to 'outside organisations' parents should give their formal consent. First of all let us assure you that we never give any commercial company the actual information that you have given us.

We do, however receive money from various companies who are anxious to know whether their products are safe. From the information you have given us on the questionnaires we are able to look at various commonly used things, from electrical appliances to foods, medicines and drinks.

If we find something worrying we will warn the company, but however helpful the money they had given us, this will not stop us from publishing the results. (ALSPAC parents newsletter, Spring 1994)

Sponsors' names and logos were not attached, as such, to any documents distributed to participants. Recognition of sponsors' contributions was acknowledged in participants' newsletters from January 1999 without involvement of the Committee. A simple list of 20 sponsors and the following statement was published: 'As we go to press the companies listed here have either sponsored a child or given us goods and services in kind'.[2] Sponsoring a child did not infer sponsorship of an individual participant, but meant that the company donated a sum that would cover the cost of a clinic visit.[3]

In 2000, another locally based company (Mail Marketing) approached Jean Golding offering to provide a liaison service between ALSPAC and commercial companies. They had suggested that some companies would pay ALSPAC to endorse their product with a logo indicating ALSPAC's approval of the product. She sought advice from the Committee, who expressed their reservations: 'respectable companies may not be as respectable as they initially seemed and it was vital [that] ALSPAC was not associated with harming children's health'. The Study mother on the Committee 'felt that ALSPAC's independence from commercial companies was of importance and valued by the study parents'.[4] It was agreed that representatives from Mail Marketing should be invited to the Committee to discuss their proposal but the company, having initially accepted, then postponed and eventually did not take up ALSPAC's offer. Collaboration with commercial companies seemed to be becoming an issue as, around the same time, it was again featured in the newsletter (see Box 8), triggered by a participant's concern.

---

### Box 8: ALSPAC study participants newsletter article

**You ask us**

*I heard that the data might be sold to companies like Coca Cola. Please tell me if this is the case or not.*
All the information collected as part of Children of the 90s belongs to the University of Bristol and is kept confidential. We do, however, accept some money from companies such as Coca Cola to look at the data. Research like this always carries a contract that says we will publish results regardless of whether the company is pleased with them or not. This is precisely the case with Coca Cola, the old British Gas (looking at the safety of gas cooking), SmithKline Beecham (looking at the safety of paracetamol), Dreamland (looking at the safety of electric blankets) and so on. Any results will be published and summarised in our newsletters. (ALSPAC parents newsletter No 19, 2000)

---

It became apparent that this article should have been worded more carefully as it was open to misinterpretation. Two thoroughly conscientious Study mothers, both of whom had completed every ALSPAC questionnaire that they had ever been sent, wrote to Jean Golding demanding to be withdrawn from the Study: 'I was disgusted … [that] you pass information on to other companies. I understand it was confidential for your research only. I feel I have been betray [sic] by this as a breach of confidentiality', and 'you insist its All Confidential. What a lot of bull'.[5] Jean Golding replied to both mothers personally, as she did to many participants who wrote to her, explaining that confidential information is never passed on to commercial companies and offering to talk to them on the phone or meet face to face if preferred. It is not clear if these mothers were persuaded to remain in the Study, but it did emphasise the importance of the guarantee of confidentiality and to the strong feelings aroused at the possibility of commercial companies obtaining personal data.

## Medical Research Council terms and conditions of grant

The issue of collaborations with commercial companies became even more pressing for the Committee in 2000 after a successful 'site visit' to ALSPAC by the Medical Research Council (MRC) and Wellcome Trust, when further substantial core funding (£5 million) for a five-year period was achieved. Jean Golding and Marcus Pembrey had first secured funding from these bodies in 1996. The two funding bodies stipulated substantial changes to several aspects of ALSPAC, including key changes to the Scientific Advisory Committee, so as to include both funders and representatives from industry. There was also much perceived pressure from the funders for 'open access' to data and encouragement to engage with commercial companies, particularly 'pharmaceutical companies concerning genetics'.[6] This did worry the Committee, who even considered asking the Vice Chancellor to get involved as 'the strict ALSPAC protocol concerning genetic analysis and refusal to sell biological samples to commercial companies may come under pressure particularly as ALSPAC will be setting up a cell-line bank with MRC funding'.[7] The Vice Chancellor's involvement was considered appropriate as all ALSPAC bio-samples (and data) were owned by the University.

By December of that year, Jean Golding had received from the MRC the terms and conditions of 'Strategic Grants awarded under the DNA collections initiative 2000'. Included in the document were a number of points. Those of most concern to the Committee were:

2. All DNA Collections in the initiative are funded on the understanding that they are to be managed as shared national resources, and must be made readily available to collaborators.…

3. Consent must be obtained from sample donors to allow the samples and associated data to be used for a range of genetic projects. Donors should be aware that samples will be part of a shared resource for use by scientists other than the team

collecting them, and that this might include scientists from commercial companies....

5. Commercial access. All requests for access by commercial companies should be referred to the MRC and the MRC should approve the terms and conditions under which such access is granted. No single company will be given exclusive access to samples collected under this initiative. Under no circumstances can the samples be sold for profit, although recovery of reasonable costs is acceptable. (Committee papers, December 2000)

Jean Golding sought advice from the Committee, as recorded in the minutes of December 2000:

The MRC document 'Terms and Conditions of Awards' was reviewed. J.G. informed the committee that the MRC would not give ALSPAC a grant until their conditions had been agreed.... She was concerned that point 2 implied collaborating with scientists whose probity was not necessarily assured and in view of the MRC's particular interest in pharmaceutical companies, she emphasised the need for ALSPAC to somehow distance itself from that position. She reminded the committee that ALSPAC has a strict protocol concerning the analysis of DNA; collaborators feedback DNA results, which are linked and analysed in our offices by ALSPAC statisticians working closely with the collaborators.

The committee agreed that the conditions were unsatisfactory particularly as they went against the guarantees we had already given to our study parents and the MRC needed to be informed of that. It was suggested that the MRC might have to change its terms and conditions in the near future depending on the recommendations from the House of Lords select committee. (Committee minutes, December 2000)

ALSPAC seemed to be in some difficulty now; core funding was, of course, essential for the continuation of the Study, especially as the funding was for the creation of cell lines (immortalised DNA), yet to comply with the terms and conditions would be breaking the guarantees given to participants when they had signed the consent forms. The Committee chose to invite representatives from the MRC to attend the Committee in order to discuss the dilemma. This involved much preparation, with several lengthy meetings to prepare ALSPAC's case. At the meeting in May 2001, attended by Dr Catherine Moody, MRC Programme Manager, 'responsible' for ALSPAC, and Dr Frances Rawle, MRC Strategic Projects Manager, responsible for the development and coordination of strategy related to DNA collections, Michael Furmston expressed the Committee's general unease at the suggestion that commercial companies would have access to ALSPAC data. Jean Golding explained how ALSPAC maintained control of genetic data: genotyping was carried out by collaborators but linkage to other ALSPAC data and statistical analyses were carried out by ALSPAC statisticians or by collaborators working in-house with these statisticians. Commercial companies had not been interested in collaborating on this basis. The Committee's anxieties seemed completely unfounded as the MRC representatives reassured the Committee that '... the conditions were written for newly funded studies and not necessarily relevant to ALSPAC. The guidelines stated the principles but were open to intelligent interpretation. Dr Moody stated that ALSPAC's procedure for peer review and ethical approval were entirely reasonable.'[8]

It is possible that a quick phone call could have resolved these issues satisfactorily but it is more likely that the painstaking preparation[9] and detailed analysis of ALSPAC's position by Michael Furmston, Jean Golding and Marcus Pembrey, plus the contributions from the Study mothers and other Committee members, left little room for any other response from the MRC.[10] The Committee was asked to adapt the terms and conditions to suit ALSPAC and, eventually, the MRC adapted its guidelines to accommodate longitudinal epidemiological studies (MRC, 2005).

## Genetic Knowledge Park

In 2001, the Committee reviewed another ambitious attempt to secure funding in collaboration with other Bristol scientists from two government departments seeking bids for a 'Genetic Knowledge Park'. This proposed 'cyber-park' was intended not only to facilitate research, but also to disseminate information to the National Health Service (NHS) and the general public. The strength of the Bristol bid was seen as ALSPAC's emphasis on health, not disease, and its progressive approach to the ethics of genetic research, as seen by the existence of the Committee and the involvement of parents in ethical decisions.[11] Crucially for the Committee, the Genetics Park would 'help local and national researchers, both academic *and commercial*, harness this unique national resource to discover the determinants of common diseases'.[12] When asked by one of the Study mothers on the Committee if this would include drug companies, Jean Golding thought that it probably would but emphasised that the 'ALSPAC protocol dictated all research using our data had to be of academic value and not conducted for profit only'.[13] The bid failed but was seen as a worthwhile exercise as it had generated useful contacts both within the University and externally.[14]

## Phenome scan

By 2002, Jean Golding, Marcus Pembrey and Richard Jones (ALSPAC Head of Biological Collections) had designed a highly original method of using ALSPAC data, which they thought might be of great interest to commercial companies. This was the 'phenome scan', which was described as 'a new approach to genotype/phenotype association studies ... in which dense phenotypic information in human cohorts is scanned for associations with individual genetic variants' (Jones et al, 2005, p 264). As explained to the Committee when Jean Golding first presented them with the concept:

> This resource will enable specified genes to be related to any number of chosen variables (medical, psychological or social) in

order to identify statistical significance. For example, if a gene was identified with high cholesterol, ALSPAC could identify other associations and enable drug manufactures to take these into account when considering side effects or other benefits of a drug to lower cholesterol. (Committee minutes, 26 February 2002)

At a subsequent meeting, Jean Golding explained the necessity for the involvement of commercial companies as 'they could do biological tests but could not make population links; ALSPAC did not have the genetic knowledge necessary, or the finances, to independently gain that knowledge'.[15]

The Committee spent several meetings discussing detailed aspects of this proposal, including financial arrangements, review process, publication policy, data management and intellectual property rights, but of most concern to the Committee was how the participants would respond to this suggestion and how it should be presented to them. There was perceived to be a subtle distinction between 'allowing access to' and 'selling data' and it was suggested that money from commercial companies could be called 'sponsorship', or 'investment' rather than 'payment' and that ALSPAC 'charged for' rather than 'sold' companies data. Several members of the Committee felt that the Study parents might be anxious that their data was being exploited for commercial purposes or shareholder profits.[16]

A few months later, Richard Jones produced a thorough and clear explanation of the phenome scan, the involvement of commercial companies and, importantly, how this would add value to ALSPAC's research endeavours (see Appendix 5). This was presented to the Clinic Team Leaders as it was thought that they would have some idea as to how Study participants would react to the idea:

Funding from pharmaceutical companies – in the public interest or selling our souls? Richard Jones has written the document that follows. He would like feedback from ALSPAC staff and is particularly interested in our views of the parents' possible reactions. *Please read it before the meeting and give the subject some thought.* Richard will join us during the discussion. (ALSPAC Clinic Team Leaders meeting, June 2002)

It is not known how the staff responded to the article but no amendments were made before it was reviewed by the Committee, who suggested that it needed to be shortened and adapted for Study parents. It seems that this did not happen, but 10 months later, a brief article was published in the participants' newsletter asking what they felt about ALSPAC working with drug companies (see Figure 6). This was shown to the Committee after it had been published with no opportunity for the Committee to amend it but Jean Golding did say that their comments would be noted for a follow-up article.[17] She twice again referred to a follow-up article – a few months later[18] and the following year[19] – yet, it seems that another article did not appear. It is not known for certain why the follow-up article did not appear. It could have been overlooked or might have been because after 4,000 newsletters had been sent,[20] Jean Golding had had no responses to the first article. Eventually, one response was received that was shown to the Committee: 'Please let Professor Golding know I trust her judgement re funding from drug companies. Do what you need to do'.[21]

**Figure 6: Participants' newsletter article**

# How can knowing about our genes improve life for children in the future?

We all have a different set of genes, which act together with one another and with different parts of our environment to make us the way we are.

We know that with so many influences it will be difficult to understand how they all fit together — and this is why it has been important to have so many thousands of Children of the 90s. This enables us to look at groups of children who have the same environment (eg live by a main road) and see why some develop a disease (eg asthma) and others do not.

If we find that the children with the problem have a particular gene, then that may help researchers and

scientists understand better why some of us get the disease. That, in turn, is more likely to help the drug companies develop medicines that are better at helping or curing the problem than any that are available now.

To make sure that medicines we take in the future are more effective and have fewer side effects, it may be possible for us to start working with drug companies. You can be quite sure that we would never sell information or samples that you have given us — but we would ask the companies for a contribution towards the costs of running the study. What would you feel about this? Please send your comments or views to Professor Golding. She would love to hear from you.

◆ **You can write to Professor Golding at:-
Children of the 90s, 24 Tyndall Avenue, Bristol BS8 1TQ**

This is another example of the actions arising from the Committee's discussions not materialising, although another newsletter article would have made little difference as no pharmaceutical companies ever expressed interest in collaborating with ALSPAC in this way. The phenome scan has been used to a limited extent, mostly by Jean Golding, who has published research using this methodology (Jones et al, 2005). Collaboration with commercial companies continued as it had done from the beginning, with strict rules about publication without veto and donations, financial or in kind, being acknowledged in the newsletters with a simple list of donors.

# FOURTEEN

## Comprehensive oversight: undocumented and unacknowledged

The Committee reviewed all data collections within ALSPAC, giving them a broad perspective of the Study as a whole. Other than Jean Golding, few recognised the importance of such all-encompassing oversight. This provided significant support not only for her, but also for the protection of the participants (always the Committee's foremost priority). None of the other ALSPAC advisory committees were aware of the detail of all that was being asked of Study participants, whether by questionnaire or in research clinics, not only in whole-cohort studies, but also in pilot studies and sub-studies, of which there were many. When the Local Research Ethics Committee (LREC) expressed concern about the amount that participants were being asked to do, with the possibility of preventing the implementation of some sub-studies, it was the ALSPAC Ethics and Law Committee who shaped Jean's robust and effective response to the LREC. Questioned by one ALSPAC Committee member of the necessity of reviewing studies in so much detail, Michael Furmston was clear that it was only by this attention to detail that the Committee was able to effectively fulfil its function.

The review of data collection proposals was central to the ALSPAC Ethics and Law Committee's unstated remit. As the extent and range of data collected by ALSPAC increased, so did the Committee's workload. On occasions when planning for a particularly intense period of data collection, such as a new research clinic, the Committee would meet four or five times within a period of six weeks. For most of the Committee, who gave up their time voluntarily and fitted the Committee's work around busy professional schedules, this was too much. One long-standing member of the Committee, David Jewell, felt that he "didn't really understand how this was an ethics committee since it seemed to be spending an awful lot of time lost in detail and very little time thinking about higher principles".[1] This was dismissed sympathetically but swiftly by the Chair with 'the devil is in the detail'[2] and, as recalled by David Jewell, "that it was only by attention to detail that we could exercise our function properly".[3]

Collaborating scientists who wished to have new data collected submitted their proposals to the Committee. Some were asked to attend Committee meetings to provide further explanation but it could be difficult for those not based locally to be in Bristol for a brief attendance at a Committee meeting. Irritatingly for the Committee, they found themselves asking collaborators for almost identical changes to a variety of different documents over the years, such as including a confidentiality clause on information sheets. It would have been beneficial to apply a more formalised pre-submission review by someone knowledgeable of the Committee's requirements to minimise these repetitive specifications. Jean Golding did view most paperwork before submission, as did the author in her capacity as Committee Secretary from 1999, but formalised and consistent pre-submission review took some years to evolve. Templates for documents such as information sheets or consent forms were not practical with such a variety of data collections within ALSPAC. The National Health Service (NHS) LRECs did introduce templates for documents such as consent forms but ALSPAC struggled to make use of them when applying for ethical approval to these committees as they were not designed for local, longitudinal population studies. Follow-up of the Committee's recommendations was not formalised either; the Committee assumed that Jean Golding would ensure that they were carried out, which, apart from occasional oversights documented elsewhere, they were.

The Committee was acutely aware of the demands being asked of the Cohort participants and continually assessed the value of the project against the burden on participants. They would consider whether it was possible to conduct the research on another population as the efficient infrastructure of ALSPAC could easily be exploited. The Scientific Advisory Committee, who reviewed research before it came to the Ethics Committee, took this factor into consideration also, so it was only occasionally that the Ethics Committee rejected research on these grounds, such as with a proposed sub-study of children with cerebral palsy: "this research did not necessarily need to make use of ALSPAC data or participants. The 36 children with cerebral palsy were already known to the health service and the additional controls could be drawn from the population at large".[4]

## Pilot studies

Pilot studies were an important aspect of ALSPAC's methodology and the Committee were given results if relevant to their review. On other occasions, if the Committee was concerned about a particular measure or set of questions, it would ask for a pilot study to be conducted and postpone their decision until the results were known. As early as their third meeting in July 1990, the Committee asked for a pilot on a questionnaire containing sensitive questions about participants' early sexual experiences. This resulted in a warning being included in the questionnaire immediately before this set of questions as the pilot participants were disturbed by the questions coming 'out of the blue'. For this first pilot study, it was suggested that before the pregnant (non-ALSPAC) mothers were approached, 'approval from the Ethics Committee be sought'.[5] This referred to the LREC as the ALSPAC Committee regarded itself as an advisory committee at that time. It appears that such approval was not obtained.

ALSPAC pilot studies continued to be conducted without ethical approval from any committee, including the ALSPAC Committee, who frequently only knew of them if results were presented. As the LRECs became more established and formalised, it was stipulated that pilot studies had to be approved before they were implemented. The ALSPAC Committee chose to ignore these requirements, believing that approval from the LRECs was not mandatory, although they continued to seek ethical approval from these NHS committees for the annual research clinics.[6] As described in Chapter Four, the bureaucracy and length of time to gain LREC approval was becoming difficult for all medical researchers, not just ALSPAC. If, as the Committee members believed, LREC approval was not obligatory, it was justifiable for the pilot studies not to be subjected to the LRECs for approval. It would be less contentious if all pilot studies had been reviewed by the Committee, but as this was not the case, it left staff and participants involved in a few pilot studies somewhat vulnerable.

## Questionnaires

Understanding the longitudinal changes taking place within the cohort was crucial to this type of epidemiological research and successive questionnaires would often have the same questions included. The Committee evolved a system of being alerted to those questions repeated from previous questionnaires and not needing to be reviewed again. However, they did insist on seeing the whole questionnaire to ensure that the length and layout were appropriate, for example, questions on self-harm or bullying were not placed at the end of the questionnaire as this could leave participants feeling unduly negative. It was a persistent challenge to find the balance between scientists' requirements for thorough and comprehensive longitudinal data without overburdening participants with lengthy and repetitive questionnaires, thus risking a rise in attrition rates.

## Research clinics

Review of the annual research clinics (Focus Clinics) constituted much of the Committee's workload. The implementation of these clinics was a considerable administrative achievement, with overlapping clinics as the cohort were born over a two-year period. Over 8,000 children attended the seven years clinic, with over 6,000 attending the 12 and 13 years clinics. It was a considerable achievement for the Ethics Committee too, who, on occasions, had to meet many times over a period of weeks in order to review all protocols, information sheets, consent forms, letters of invitation, reminders and letters to GPs.

## Blood samples

The method of taking blood from children attending the Children in Focus clinics came under scrutiny as, in the early 1990s, there was:

> ... considerable pressure to transfer blood testing from the group of procedures designated to pose 'no risk' into the 'low risk' category. Although such a proposal had recently been rejected by the BPA [British Paediatric Association] ... other ethics committees had been considering whether it was in the interests of healthy children to be given blood tests for the purpose of research. (Committee minutes, May 1992)

The 'pressure' referred to in the minutes came from guidelines issued by not only the BPA in 1992 (BPA, 1992), but also both the Royal College of Physicians in 1990 (RCP, 1990) and the Medical Research Council in 1991 (MRC, 1991).

By 1994, when the 'Children in Focus' were approaching two years old, the Committee were asked to consider blood sampling by venepuncture rather than heel pricks, which had been the method used at previous clinics. There was lengthy discussion about the potential distress caused when taking blood by various methods: heel prick, finger prick or venepuncture. A pilot study was conducted to assess if distress could be minimised or eliminated during venepuncture, as discussed by Elizabeth Mumford (1999a). Members of the Committee watched the testing in progress and agreed to permit venepuncture using anaesthetic cream and a fine butterfly needle, with only one attempt to obtain blood and, most importantly, the assent of the child. This, plus the addition of a 'Postman Pat' or similar video that was viewed during the procedure, worked remarkably well. At the final 'Children in Focus' clinic when the children were approximately five years old and venepuncture had been used at two previous clinics, 81% of parents gave permission for venepuncture, with samples obtained from 82% of these (that is 66% of the attendees).[7]

## Sub-studies

It was only in the last month of Michael Furmston's 16-year period as Chair of the Ethics Committee that formal terms of reference for the Committee were formulated. These were minimal (see Chapter One) and gave no indication of the Committee's commitment to reviewing the details of data collection. Slightly more indication of the Committee's broader remit had been documented within the web-based protocol in 2001[8] (see Box 9) but the stated 'detailed scrutiny of all aspects of the study', including the 'Ethics of Nested Studies' (sub-studies), evolved over time.

---

### Box 9: The ALSPAC Ethics and Law Committee

The ALSPAC Ethics and Law Committee was set up in 1989 before the study children were born and while many pilot studies were being conducted in order to advise on the ethical and legal aspects of the study. This independent committee, chaired by a lawyer, has broad membership: medical ethicist, two study mothers, legal medical expert, philosopher, paediatrician, GP, child psychiatrist, head teacher and school health nurse. The Committee meets every month and insists on rigorous and detailed scrutiny of all aspects of the study. This includes:

- Data: Questionnaires, Hands-on Measurements and Biological Samples.
- Confidentiality and Anonymity.
- Consent and Assent.
- Ethics of Nested Studies.
- Individual Feedback: Prospective and Retrospective.
- Child Protection, Staff Protection and Data Protection.

---

Although Jean Golding's intention was for the Committee to review all sub-studies involving new data collections, this was not always the case. An update of sub-studies was presented to the Committee in 1999[9] but not all had been reviewed in detail prior to the start of the studies (nitrogen oxide and carbon monoxide studies, stepfamilies study and an alcohol and breastfeeding study). Two months earlier, Jean Golding had received a letter from one of the LREC Chairs expressing concern at the intensity of the data collection:

… the Committee [LREC] has become increasingly concerned that consent given to the initial longitudinal study has been extrapolated to the continuation of that study, and that the involvement of the subjects had become increasingly intense. The subjects, having invested considerable time in the on-going study in its previous forms may feel more obliged to continue participation than would otherwise be the case.

Of even greater concern is the use of the same population of subjects in satellite projects, the database of which appears to be given or sold to other researchers so that the subject population can be contacted again and involved in yet further studies, disruption of school, and time off work for the parent. Despite assurances, it does take an effort of will to refuse to participate in such studies.

If the index subjects of all these diverse studies are the same in each case, over-exposure to research is taking place. If the controls of such studies are the same in more than one satellite study it is probable that over-exposure is taking place. The Committee needs assurance that persuasion, even coercion, however politely applied, is not being exerted unethically to make these studies, albeit valuable possible. We realise that the information gathered on this subject population is extremely valuable and it would be far more inconvenient to gather such a wealth of data on any other subject population. Yet, the interests of the subject must be considered before and above the interests of the research. (Committee papers, December 1998)

Jean Golding showed the ALSPAC Committee the letter and a robust response was formulated:

- Response rates are still high (78% of those invited attended the Focus at 7 clinics).
- Postal invitations do not pressurise participants in the way that a face-to-face interview or telephone call might.
- Pilot studies were conducted in order to ascertain how participants would respond to further testing.
- Participants are only selected if they had not taken part in a previous sub-study (as either a case or control). This policy could not be implemented by other research studies in the Bristol area.
- Lists of participants are never given or sold to other researchers.
- The Scientific Advisory Committee assesses whether each new proposal needs to make use of ALSPAC data (Ethics Committee may also reject a proposal on these grounds).

There is no record of the LREC meeting or how the response was received. Sub-studies continued to be included within ALSPAC and reviewed by the Committee (see Box 10).

## Box 10: Sub-study topics reviewed by the ALSPAC Ethics and Law Committee

- Activity
- Adult learning
- Air pollution
  - ◊ Volatile organic compounds
  - ◊ Carbon monoxide
  - ◊ Nitrogen dioxide
- Allergy
- Anaemia
- Antisocial behaviour
- Asthma
- Bunk bed sharing
- Cholesterol
- Cognition
- Complementary and alternative medicines
- Cortisol
- Day care
- Developmental impairments
- Diet
- Electromagnetic fields
- Ethics (participants' perspectives)

- Fingerprints
- Fitness
- Fractures
- Growth
- Hearing
- Laterality
- Lead
- Lesbian families
- Lung function
- Memory
- Miscarriage
- Noise
- Nursery thermometers
- Peanut allergy
- Pesticides
- Radon
- Skin
- Speech
- Stress
- Teeth
- Twins' language
- Vision

## Comprehensive oversight

The importance of the Committee's painstaking review of all data collected by ALSPAC, whether by questionnaire, in research clinics or within the many sub-studies, was evaluated by David Jewell, who said:

"[The Committee] has considered, advised on and approved most of the studies and data collection that go on in ALSPAC and that involves very familiar principles of research ethics – of consent, risks and benefits, confidentiality, duty of care and things like that – and ALSPAC developed a certain expertise, particularly on confidentiality. The ... thing which just emerged out of the consideration of all the studies is therefore [that the Committee] had an oversight of the study as a whole." (David Jewell, Oral History Interview, 2012)

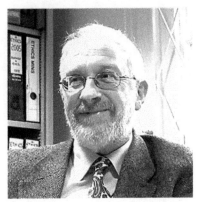

David Jewell

This he admitted had not become clear to him until he had been a member of the Committee for over a decade. None of the other ALSPAC Committees that also had broad remits, such as the Steering Committee or Scientific Advisory Committee, reviewed all aspects of ALSPAC in such thorough detail. Other than Jean Golding, there were no others who had a grasp of both the detail and a wider perspective of the Study. The recognition of the importance of such all-encompassing oversight was rarely, if ever, acknowledged or documented.

# FIFTEEN

## Influence beyond ALSPAC: extension of expertise

The Committee's influence became considerably wider than just ALSPAC as its groundbreaking work became known. There were formal consultations not only by policymakers such as House of Lords Science and Technology Sub-Committee and the European Society of Human Genetics, but also by many other national and international cohort studies. Beyond the formal consultations, ALSPAC was an exemplar for other cohort studies and Jean Golding and her staff provided much informal guidance, without many realising how the Committee's sound legal and ethical advice had underpinned the Study from the very beginning.

On several occasions, the ALSPAC Ethics and Law Committee were asked their advice by various national and international organisations. As the first ethics committee dealing with issues arising from the collection of genetic material from a population sample, advice on genetic issues was of particular importance. Although Marcus Pembrey was not a member of the Ethics Committee, as ALSPAC's Director of Genetics, he was well aware of the Committee's work and was involved with influential national and international policymaking bodies. He was consulted by the Committee if advice was sought on issues ranging from DNA banking and data storage to consent and confidentiality.

The Committee was seen as an example for other cohort studies at a time when there were few guidelines and little interest in the ethical issues raised by longitudinal birth cohorts such as ALSPAC by the National Health Service (NHS) Local Research Ethics Committees.

## European Society of Human Genetics

In 1999, Marcus Pembrey asked Michael Furmston and the Committee to contribute to *Guidelines on data storage and DNA banking for biomedical research* (Godard et al, 2003), which was being developed by the Professional and Public Policy Committee (PPPC) of the European Society of Human Genetics. The PPPC was, in effect, the Society's ethics committee[1] and was simultaneously drafting guidelines on Insurance and Employment, Genetic Screening, and Genetic Services.[2] Professor Pembrey emphasised that the PPPC '... particularly want to learn from, and analyse, real examples of how professionals have tackled the issues raised by DNA banking.... [and] wish to include two contrasting examples of genetic epidemiology – ALSPAC and the proposed commercial deCODE healthcare database in Iceland.'[3] The issues that the PPPC identified for debate were:

- consent requirements for banking and further use of human genetic material;
- protection of confidentiality;
- control and ownership;
- access to and sharing of banked samples;
- duration of storage and withdrawal of samples;
- regulatory mechanisms of banking.

Michael Furmston and John Henderson (paediatrician and member of the Committee) attended a meeting in Paris, which brought together a total of 50 experts from 12 European countries from a diversity of backgrounds involved with DNA banking. The subsequent paper was reviewed by the ALSPAC Committee before publication (Godard et al, 2003).

## House of Lords Science and Technology Sub-Committee

In July 2000, Jean Golding received an invitation from the House of Lords Science and Technology Sub-Committee to submit a written contribution for their Inquiry into Human Genetic Databases. This inquiry was to focus on 'current activity … [as] future regulatory requirements will be addressed by the Human Genetics Commission'[4] at a later date. Four years later, the Human Genetics Commission also consulted the ALSPAC Ethics and Law Committee, although with some ambivalence, as will be seen. The questions that the Sub-Committee asked were extensive:

1. What current projects involve collecting genetic information on people in the UK? What other projects are about to start? Are there collections of material (eg tissue samples) that could be used to generate databases of DNA profiles?
2. Why are these genetic databases being assembled? How are these activities funded? What practical considerations will constrain developments? Are there alternative ways of fulfilling the objectives?
3. What is the genetic information that is being collected? How is it being stored and protected?
4. How do the organisations involved see their responsibilities regarding privacy, consent, future use, public accountability and intellectual property rights?
5. How do they see their activities in the area of genetic databases developing in the future? What advances in sequencing, screening and database technology are they anticipating?
6. What lessons should be learnt from genetic database initiatives in other countries?

The call for evidence noted that 'It is recognised that individual witnesses may feel able to address only some of these [questions] … [therefore] evidence is expected principally from the bodies which are involved in maintaining, developing or using human genetic databases'. ALSPAC and one other UK longitudinal study (the North

Cumbrian Community Genetics Project) were asked to submit evidence, although ALSPAC was 'used as an example of excellent practice in other submissions including those from the Wellcome Trust and MRC'.[5] The other organisations approached to submit evidence were an amorphous and extremely wide-ranging group, all apparently 'maintaining, planning or using human genetic databases' (see Figure 7).

**Figure 7: Inquiry into Human Genetic Databases consultees**

**INQUIRY INTO *HUMAN GENETIC DATABASES***
Bodies (or their representative organisations) which may be maintaining, planning or using human genetic databases (as defined) to which the call for evidence in this Inquiry is being sent

The UK Health Departments and respective parts of the NHS
The Medicines Control Agency
The Medical Devices Agency
The Human Fertilisation and Embryology Authority
Home Office
The Forensic Science Service
Association of Chief Police Officers in England, Wales and Northern Ireland
Association of Chief Police Officers in Scotland
The Data Protection Commissioner
Child Support Agency
x North Cumbria Community Genetics Project
x Avon Longitudinal Study of Parents and Children
Office of Science and Technology
Biotechnology and Biological Sciences Research Council
Medical Research Council
Wellcome Trust
The Association of Medical Research Charities
British Heart Foundation
Imperial Cancer Research Fund
Cancer Research Campaign
Royal Society
Royal Pharmaceutical Society
Academy of Medical Royal Colleges
Academy of Medical Sciences
General Medical Council
General Dental Council

UKCC for Nursing etc
The Academy of Medical Sciences
Association of British Insurers
The Association of the British Pharmaceutical Industry
BioIndustry Association
Glaxo Wellcome
SmithKline Beecham
Astra Zeneca
Pfizer
Eli Lilly
Novartis
Roche
British Biotech
Sanger Centre
European Bioinformatics Institute
European Agency for the Evaluation of Medicinal Products
UNESCO
WHO
Key contacts in:
    Estonia
    France
    Iceland
    Japan
    Sweden
    Ukraine
    USA

The written submission approved by the Committee was entirely descriptive (see Box 11),[6] unlike the written evidence submitted by Marcus Pembrey some years later to the Genomic Medicine Science and Technology Committee. Professor Pembrey cites his 'relevant expertise' as ALSPAC's Director of Genetics among many other prestigious posts and refers to the work of the ALSPAC Ethics Committee. It makes for entertaining reading as he does not hold back in his criticism of the Wellcome Trust's 'disproportionate influence on policy' and their 'naïve' understanding of issues of wide access to data when related to ongoing cohort studies.[7]

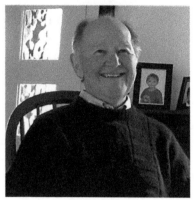

Marcus Pembrey

---

**Box 11: Summary of written submission to the House of Lords Science and Technology Sub-Committee**

- Extraction of DNA included in the methodology from the beginning.
- Information given to Study mothers, including no feedback of genetic analyses.
- Governance of the Study, with list of advisory committees.
- Funding, including from commercial companies.
- Analysis of samples only with written consent (even if collected without consent through NHS sources).
- Recognition of limitations of DNA stock, especially with the advance of the human genome project, and therefore investigation into immortalised cell lines.
- Consent.
- Collaboration and methods of preserving anonymity.

---

## Joint Human Genetics Commission and National Screening Committee

In 2003, again through Marcus Pembrey's connections, the Joint Human Genetics Commission (HGC) and National Screening Committee (NSC) officially visited the ALSPAC Ethics and Law Committee. The HGC was a prestigious non-departmental public body that advised the Government on ethical and social aspects of a variety of genetic issues. At the time, it was chaired by Baroness Helena Kennedy QC and included Sir John Sulston and other highly esteemed individuals. It was disbanded in 2010 after the new Government's review of all government quangos. The NSC role was to advise ministers and the NHS on aspects of population screening. The two committees had formed a joint sub-committee as they intended '… to consult both the public and ALSPAC experts about the feasibility and ethics of obtaining DNA samples from all children in the U.K. at birth. They had expressed interest in meeting members of the ALSPAC ethics committee, particularly the Study mothers.'[8]

Prior to the HGC/NSC sub-committee visit, the author and Marcus Pembrey were invited to attend a meeting in London to briefly discuss and plan the visit. At this meeting, one of the sub-committee expressed incomprehension as to why they should be consulting the ALSPAC Committee. It appeared that they did not feel that ALSPAC or the Ethics Committee had much to offer them. The two-day visit went ahead despite these reservations, with the University of Bristol's Vice Chancellor himself hosting a dinner for both Committees in one of the University's most attractive buildings, the 18th-century Royal Fort House. It was reported by the ALSPAC Committee members who attended this dinner that copious quantities of alcohol were consumed that evening. This might not be entirely irrelevant as the following day, the brief presentations given by Marcus Pembrey, Michael Furmston, Jean Golding and Alastair Campbell (Professor of Ethics in Medicine and member of the ALSPAC Committee) seemed to fall quite flat. Marcus Pembrey had recommended that the 'presentations [should be] kept fairly short as members of the Commission tend to like to ask lots of questions and have time for more general discussions'.[9] There were, in fact, few questions and minimal discussion despite the relevance of the material presented, particularly by Marcus, who described ALSPAC's contribution to developments in genetic screening/profiling. Perhaps it had been correct to assume that the ALSPAC Committee had nothing to contribute or possibly the dearth of questions was due to the Vice Chancellor's lavish hospitality the previous night. However, Jean Golding reported to the ALSPAC Committee '... that she had had some unofficial feedback from John Sulston. The subcommittee's report at the end of the year would recommend to the government that adequate funding for studies like ALSPAC were vital if genetic screening at birth is to be beneficial.'[10]

## UK Biobank and the Nuffield Trust

UK Biobank, the longitudinal study that recruited 500,000 individuals nationwide aged between 40 and 69 during 2006–10, has many similarities to ALSPAC despite being national, much larger and only recruiting adults of a certain age. The study had a lengthy period of planning and consultation, including producing an Ethics and Governance Framework (EGF) to 'set standards for the project, and to ensure that safeguards are in place for scientifically and ethically approved research'.[11] The draft EGF was developed in 2003 by a small Interim Advisory Committee chaired by Dr William Lowrance, a well-respected international consultant in health policy and ethics. The previous year, William Lowrance had led workshops for the Nuffield Trust on a variety of issues, culminating in the publication of *Learning from experience: Privacy and the secondary use of data in health research* (Lowrance, 2002). It was at one of these workshops that Dr Lowrance, much to his surprise, discovered that ALSPAC had been collecting genetic material from a population sample for over a decade. In November 2004, the UK Biobank set up an independent Ethics and Governance Council (EGC), chaired by Professor Alastair Campbell, to oversee adherence to the EGF. Professor Campbell was not only the University of Bristol's first Director of the Centre for Ethics in Medicine (founded in June 1998), but had also been a member of the ALSPAC Ethics and Law Committee from 1996 for several years.

There is some confusion as to how much the ALSPAC Committee's deliberations on the issues surrounding longitudinal genetic research influenced the UK Biobank's EGF or EGC. Gordon Stirrat, a colleague of Alastair Campbell and a long-standing member of the ALSPAC Ethics and Law Committee, reported in October 2004, one month prior to the establishment of the UK Biobank EGC, 'that he had spoken to Alastair Campbell about the Biobank Ethics Committee. Professor Campbell said that there was no analogy between that committee and the ALSPAC Law and Ethics committee'.[12] This did not deter Professor Stirrat from advising Professor Campbell to make use of the ALSPAC Committee's expertise as, six months later, Professor Stirrat reported to the ALSPAC Committee that '... Professor Campbell had recently spoken to G.S. [Gordon Stirrat] about some of the issues his committee has to consider e.g. single gene disorders. G.S. strongly advised Professor Campbell to liaise with J.G. [Jean Golding] and M.F. [Michael Furmston] as the ALSPAC Law & Ethics Committee had grappled with such issues for many years.'[13] As far as is known, Alastair Campbell did not take up this suggestion. It is clear that there were many interlinking strands between the two ethics committees (as well as between other senior members of both organisations),[14] and by 2011, Gordon Stirrat suggested that UK Biobank EGC was probably designed on the ALSPAC Committee (Overy et al, 2012, p 36).

Whatever the truth, ALSPAC influenced UK Biobank in other ways, as stated by Professor Rory Collins, Principal Investigator and Chief Executive of UK Biobank, when giving evidence to the Genomic Medicine – Science and Technology Parliamentary Committee in 2008[15]:

I believe that participation, particularly on a population-wide basis, in such studies is a great way for people to understand better what they can produce, in being part of something that will improve health. I can give you an example of this. The Wellcome Trust funded ALSPAC [which] is a study of children and mothers in Bristol. We are now recruiting into UK Biobank in Bristol and our recruitment rate there is twice as high as in any other part of the country in which we are recruiting. I cannot tell you that it is definitely because of ALSPAC, but many people who come in do talk about the ALSPAC study.

This has been termed 'the ALSPAC Effect', as described at the Society of Longitudinal and Life Course Studies international conference in 2014 (O'Hare, 2014).

## National Children's Study

The influence of the ALSPAC Committee was not restricted to the UK. When the US National Institutes of Health were planning the National Children's Study, an ill-fated nationwide longitudinal birth cohort of 100,000, an ethics workshop was held as part of a lengthy consultation process. Representatives from seven established longitudinal cohort studies were invited to present their studies, with particular emphasis on the ethical problems encountered. ALSPAC was the only non–US-based cohort represented. The influence on the subsequent ethical decisions was almost certainly negligible[16] as the minimalist approach to the feedback of results was not an accepted policy in the US at that time.

Apart from the formal consultations, when the Committee's expertise was recognised and advice actively sought, it is difficult to gauge how influential the Committee was beyond ALSPAC. It is likely that the influence was somewhat concealed. ALSPAC was an exemplar for many longitudinal studies that have since been set up and advice was frequently sought from Jean Golding and her staff on many aspects of the Study. She arranged carefully organised and much-appreciated personalised tours of ALSPAC's clinics and departments for numerous visitors. She also edited a well-received guide to longitudinal studies (Golding et al, 2009) commissioned by the World Health Organisation together with the US National Institutes of Health, based largely on her experience with ALSPAC, which included a paper on the ethics of longitudinal cohort studies (Birmingham and Doyle, 2009). Perhaps not known by those seeking advice (or those learning from ALSPAC without formal consultation) was how significant the Committee had been in influencing ALSPAC on all levels.

# Conclusions

Jean Golding believed that ALSPAC would have developed quite differently if the radical idea of the Study having its own ethics committee had not been implemented. There was no question that she valued the support of the Committee but whether the Study would have been so different without its own sound legal and ethical advice is disputed by some. The fact that there were no major ethical calamities must be in no small part due to the Committee's influence; first, establishing principles, and then producing compatible policies when presented with the real issues emerging from the Study. These were early days for research ethics committees and the style and structure of the Committee did not comply with today's idea of best practice. Computing was also in its infancy and a complex and original system known as the 'Ethical Divide' was designed to protect the Study participants' anonymity, the key principle on which the Study was founded. The Committee was aware of the pioneering nature of its own work and was not only willing to advise a variety of influential organisations, but also supported academic publications that described its method and impact. Pragmatic solutions to the myriad of ethical issues were found at a time when there were no governance structures in place for medical research of any kind, let alone a study of ALSPAC's ambition and complexity.

The success of the ALSPAC Ethics and Law Committee as a supportive, advisory group to the Director is evident from Jean Golding's own account. Apart from the meetings being "a joy", which is almost certainly the only time meetings of a research ethics committee have been described as such, she credited the Committee with much of ALSPAC's success: "From my point of view, the importance was [that] this body of opinion and advice … was there, meeting every month or so, without which I don't think ALSPAC would have developed in the way it did at all".[1] Although too modest to articulate how it did develop, others are less reticent. The 'Jean Golding Institute for data-intensive research' within the University of Bristol, established in 2016, states on its website[2]:

The Institute is named after Jean Golding OBE, Emeritus Professor of Paediatric and Perinatal Epidemiology and founder of the Avon Longitudinal Study of Parents and Children (ALSPAC or Children of the Nineties). For over two decades this ground breaking study of over 14,000 pregnant women and their children has given world-leading insight into the environmental and genetic factors that affect human development – and shown the power of using data-intensive research to improve people's lives.

Committee members will testify to the research being 'data-intensive', having developed a remit of comprehensive oversight and having reviewed nearly all the primary data collections in detail over many years. The 'world leading insights' have been recognised also, as is evident by the World Health Organisation commissioning Jean Golding to write *A guide to undertaking a Birth cohort study: Purposes, pitfalls and practicalities* (Golding et al, 2009), which included a chapter on ethics and governance (Birmingham and Doyle, 2009). The influence of the Committee on the whole Study is difficult to quantify. David Baum and others on the Steering Committee recognised the importance of the ethical dimensions of such an ambitious longitudinal study and therefore instigated an Ethics and Law Committee attached to the Study itself – an entirely new concept. Their grasp of the ethical issues significantly influenced the design of the Study so as to include the principle of anonymity and broad consent for the use of genetic material prior to the Ethics and Law Committee's involvement. Richard Ashcroft considered the impact of the Ethics and Law Committee on the Study as a whole when interviewed in 2013:

"... what made ALSPAC work wasn't getting high-quality ethical advice from a committee, it was a very well-conceived study, very well organised with very strong clear leadership and an extremely good relationship with its participants and the wider community and if any of those things hadn't been in place, then no matter how good its Ethics Committee was, it would have failed. And if you take the Ethics Committee out of that picture, well, who knows what difference that would have made? I think it did make a difference, certainly at the outset, and there were probably certain key moments in the history of ALSPAC where it did play a critical role." (Richard Ashcroft, Oral History Interview, 2013)

One of the key moments at the outset was captured in David Baum's memo when he wrote of 'establishing the absolute principle of non-attributability' (see Figure 1 in Chapter One), that is, the anonymisation, or more precisely pseudo-anonymisation, as longitudinal and other data linkage was essential to the Study. This was embedded in the Study methodology alongside 'Consent', the other key principle identified by Michael Fursmston at the very first Committee meeting. The principle of non-attributability had to be incorporated into all the Committee's evolving policies, such as child protection, the disclosure of individual results or linkage to external databases, although Michael Furmston was quite clear that it was the Committee's remit to decide if and when, in specific circumstances, this principle should be disregarded.

As promised to the Study participants on enrolment, 'a very complicated set of procedures' had to be designed to incorporate this principle in order to 'ensure that no one will be able to link the information that you give us with your name'.[3] This was in 1990 when computers were in their infancy and were only just being introduced into offices throughout the country. The implementation of this fundamental ethical principle stipulated by the Committee, known variously as the 'Ethical Divide' or the 'Golden Rule', fell to David

Carmichael, the ALSPAC Data Manger. When asked about the origins of the 'Ethical Divide' in 2016, he stated with characteristic modesty:

I don't claim to have invented the Divide, at all. The original specification for ALSPAC said (I paraphrase) that no-one would be able to pick up a questionnaire and link that back to a real person nor link contents from one questionnaire to another, except anonymously. My interpretation was quite literal, hence the myriad of IDs, one for each collection point.... The protocol also stated that person data (name, address, etc.) would not be stored on the same computer as research data. At the start that was simple to enforce, but I knew that networking, which was really just beginning then, would make this unlikely to be sustainable. Hence the overkill of a separate ID per collection point. This I wouldn't do now, but it was a new aspect of data collection that had really [never] been dealt with [before]. (David Carmichael, personal correspondence, November 2016)

Although eventually abandoned as too cumbersome, credit must be given to David Carmichael for establishing 'the Divide' and, with it, not only the application of the Committee's principles, but also an ethos within the staff group of respect for confidentiality and an understanding of the principle of anonymity guaranteed to the Cohort. Trust in the researchers' integrity by the Study participants had to be established rapidly if the Study was to succeed. As a large local study, Cohort families were everywhere, including within the staff group itself, and any breach of the guarantee could have had disastrous repercussions.

As it transpired, there were no major catastrophes, which must be in no small part due to the Committee's influence; first, establishing principles, and then producing compatible policies when presented with the real issues emerging from the Study, while gradually taking on the unacknowledged oversight of ALSPAC's activities. There were inconsistencies, omissions and some harsh decisions when trying to adhere to the principles but they were dealing with rapidly evolving research with few established guidelines.

The structure of research ethics committees was also not established and the ALSPAC Ethics and Law Committee certainly did not conform to current practice as to how a committee should be set up and conducted:

- Committee members themselves questioned how independent they could or should be, even when they acquired Institutional Review Board registration in the US and, with it, formal change in status from advisory to independent. Jean Golding was encouraged to continue on the Committee after her retirement and her status as a 'non-voting member' seemed entirely inconsequential.

- For Study participants to serve as full members of the Committee was regarded as progressive and appropriate by some at the time. Having 'service users' or 'stakeholders' involved in research design and ethics is becoming almost mandatory nowadays, although UK Biobank's Ethics and Governance Council does not replicate this practice as it is thought that it might compromise their independence.

- New Committee members were chosen through informal recommendation by other Committee members or those known to them, resulting in the similarity of members, who were all white, middle-class professionals. Jean Golding favoured membership by invitation as she thought advertising for members attracted individuals with an 'axe to grind'. She was quite prepared to take risks, though, and invited onto the Committee one impressive and subsequently long-standing member who was initially recommended with the qualification that they were 'a bit of a maverick'.

- Terms of reference did not exist until just before Michael Furmston retired as Chair. He retrospectively articulated the remit of the Committee that had been established over the previous 16 years in the broadest possible terms, with a succinct 60 words.

- Minutes were sometimes intentionally embellished and although Elizabeth Mumford and the author endeavoured to ensure that they were not misleading in any way, Michael Furmston once cheerfully held that Elizabeth Mumford documented what should have been said, not necessarily what was said.
- The Chair remained in situ for 16 years and many other Committee members served for well over a decade. This was vital to the Committee's method of working as, otherwise, in Gordon Stirrat's words, 'some of the folk memory would be lost'.
- The informality and affability between Committee members, appreciated by many as essential in facilitating open and honest discussion, however difficult the issues, was considered by some, both then and now, as too casual.

As Tim Chambers reflected when remembering his time on the Committee:

> "There was a serious core to it, but it was slightly, sort of, well, 'we'll get some good brains together and we'll chew this through' [but] as a first ethics committee in the University, how [else] do you get these things started?"[4]

A major part of the 'serious core' and crucial to the Committee's work was the legal guidance from the two lawyers on the Committee. There was little in English law specifically related to medical research of any kind, let alone observational studies such as ALSPAC. Michael Furmston and Elizabeth Mumford were always mindful that they might have to defend the Committee's decisions in court. They therefore ensured that they always had confidence that any ruling on a decision would most likely be in ALSPAC's favour. They were never put to that particular test.

The Committee, aware of the pioneering nature of their work, supported academic undertakings concerning their own methodology and impact. Alastair Campbell, a member of the Committee and Professor of Medical Ethics, brought one such academic initiative before the Committee in 1994. He suggested a study of the Committee's decision-making, based on the Committee minutes and referring to the literature in the area. This was considered too similar to work already under way by Elizabeth Mumford but the Committee welcomed his suggestion of a comparison between the ALSPAC Committee and other comparable committees. It is not clear how many other comparable committees there were nationally or internationally, but, unfortunately, the study did not materialise. Elizabeth Mumford went on to publish two papers (Mumford, 1999a, 1999b), which were well received by both the Committee and the Local Research Ethics Committees.

The Committee's interests went beyond their own work, however, and in 1999, Richard Ashcroft proposed a study, designed by himself, Marcus Pembrey and some of the other Committee members, 'investigating the perceptions of adult and child participants about the ethical safeguards adopted for their protection'.[5] The methodology of this proposal developed into a far more independent investigation than originally suggested, and apart from Richard Ashcroft, all Committee members withdrew from any active participation in the Study. This prestigious three-year qualitative study,[6] funded by the Wellcome Trust, not only deprived the Committee of Richard Ashcroft, who resigned due to a conflict of interest as he remained one of the principal investigators, but also put considerable strain on the relationship between his staff and the ALSPAC staff, including the author. He stated several times in his interview that "It was the most difficult piece of research I have ever done". He also reflected that "In hindsight, it was a mixture of entirely understandable caution on the part of ALSPAC itself and Jean Golding in person, and a feeling that a very inexperienced junior, slightly hot-headed researcher, that is to say, me, could jeopardise things."[7] Despite the complexities of the interactions between the two staff groups, the results were of great value. Marcus Pembrey (who gave a joint presentation with one of Richard Ashcroft's staff many years later) became visibly moved when describing a Study child's concerns and how these had confirmed his long-held views:

"… their main worry was … that the doctors would get bored with analysing it all because it takes so long … and they would move on and do something else and that all this effort that they individually and collectively had given to fill in all these forms and everything else, that somehow it wouldn't be used in the future for research … and that the researchers would lose heart, give up and so on. Very insightful.… It chimed with the way I had always viewed the general public. They really are not bothered about you having all their information, and so on, yes. What they want is to cooperate and be true partners in this research and for us to not give up. And with people like Jean, you don't give up." (Marcus Pembrey, Oral History Interview, 2013)

Marcus Pembrey felt that this sub-study validated his strongly held belief that the addition of a genetic component to ALSPAC was not, at least for the Cohort participants, particularly problematic. This supposedly highly contentious aspect of the Study had, in fact, taken up very little of the Committee's time, although it came into other areas that the Committee discussed at length, such as the consent for and collection and use of biological samples or divulging individual results. The emphasis on anonymity and confidentiality, alongside the carefully nurtured trust in the integrity of Jean Golding and her researchers, almost certainly pre-empted or alleviated the anxieties of the participants in this respect.

On Michael Furmston's retirement from the Committee, Marcus Pembrey, who was a little more detached than some, having never been on the Committee, put its work into context when he wrote to him:

It is only with hindsight that one realises that ALSPAC was ground breaking in so many ways. The establishment and detailed work of the Law and Ethics Committee [sic] is a clear example. In a world of gene-hype on the one hand and anti-genetics on the other, your committee's work and judgements represent a triumph of rational policy making. Of course there have been and are tricky issues but your committee has done the careful work necessary to find sensible workable solutions. What a contrast to the knee-jerk reaction brigade! (Marcus Pembrey, 'Letter to Michael Furmston', 11 October 2007)

These insights could be applied to all of the ALSPAC Ethics and Law Committee's work, not just to the genetic component. Sensible workable solutions were found for the tricky issues despite the occasional inconsistencies. This unique, pioneering committee surely does represent a triumph of rational policymaking.

# Postscript

The Avon Longitudinal Study of Parents and Children (ALSPAC) becomes more exceptional the more one learns about it. Led by Jean Golding and later George Davey Smith, it has clearly been a study that has continued in the pursuit of research into health and disease throughout the life course from early pregnancy onwards. If we are in the business of understanding the forebears of adult disorder (or health), then this is the way to do it. However, in delivering such an overarching and comprehensive screen of health and epidemiologically relevant data, this Study has, of course, needed to remain at the forefront of ethical practice and governance. This was not easy – at least when there were no formal structures to work to, as ALSPAC encountered in the early years. Participating in science now, one is faced with a clearly defined and executable set of requirements that ensure study activity is transparent, guided in full view of the participants and appropriate. This seems somewhat of a luxury given the testing times that ALSPAC previously encountered and it is to that endeavour (for ALSPAC and other studies like it) that the current scientific community must doff its cap. In this case, the tireless energy and contributions of Professors Jean Golding, David Baum, Marcus Pembury, Michael Furmston and other important contributors (so well described in this text) present a great lesson in the delivery of ethical research but also in the difficulties and idiosyncrasies seen along the way. Long may the Study continue.

*Nicholas Timpson, Professor of Genetic Epidemiology,*
*ALSPAC Principle Investigator, August 2017*

# Notes

## Introduction

[1] See: www.bristol.ac.uk/alspac/

[2] See: www.cls.ioe.ac.uk/

[3] See: https://web-beta.archive.org/web/20030131132233/http://www.alspac.bris.ac.uk:80/AlspacExt/MainProtocol/Introduction%20and%20welcome2.htm

[4] See: www.genome.gov/10001772/all-about-the--human-genome-project-hgp/

[5] Marcus Pembrey, Oral History Interview, 2013.

[6] The UK county of Avon was abolished in 1996. It was situated 120 miles west of London on the River Severn estuary. It had a population of approximately 1 million, about half of which resided in the city of Bristol. It comprised a mixture of rural areas, inner-city deprivation, leafy suburbs and moderate-sized towns.

[7] See: http://webarchive.nationalarchives.gov.uk/+/http://www.dh.gov.uk/en/Publicationsandstatistics/Publications/PublicationsPolicyAndGuidance/DH_4002874

[8] Further information relating to confidentiality for participants if requested (ALSPAC Ethics Archive, A/90/10/08/1).

## Chapter One: Preliminaries and pioneers: framing the questions

[1] Gordon Stirrat, Oral History Interview, 2013.

[2] Elizabeth Mumford, Oral History Interview, 2013.

[3] Tim Chambers, Oral History Interview, 2013.

[4] Richard Ashcroft, Oral History Interview, 2013.

[5] Gordon Stirrat, Oral History Interview, 2013.

6  Ian Lister Cheese, Oral History Interview, 2013.
7  Committee minutes, 3 August 1993 (ALSPAC Ethics Archive, A/93/08/03/M) and 18 October 1999 (ALSPAC Ethics Archive, A/99/10/18/M).
8  Draft instructions for home interviewers (ALSPAC Ethics Archive, A/90/08/22/1/b).
9  ALSPAC data protection risk assessment: confidentiality documents, appendix 3i–x, March 2000 (author's personal archive).
10  Richard Ashcroft, Oral History Interview, 2013.
11  Ruud ter Muelen, personal correspondence, April 2011.
12  David Jewell, Oral History Interview, 2012.
13  Letter to Chair of British Paediatric Association Ethics Advisory Committee from David Baum, 18 May 1990 (ALSPAC Ethics Archive, C/90/05/18/CN/DB).
14  Letter to David Baum from Chair of British Paediatric Association Ethics Advisory Committee, 18 June 1990 (ALSPAC Ethics Archive, C/90/06/18/DB/CN).
15  Gordon Stirrat, Oral History Interview, 2013.

## Chapter Two: Informal or casual: an unusual style

1  Michael Furmston, Oral History Interview, 2012.
2  Tim Chambers, Oral History Interview, 2013.
3  Ian Lister Cheese, Oral History Interview, 2013.
4  Richard Ashcroft, Oral History Interview, 2013.
5  Jean Golding, Oral History Interview, 2012.
6  Richard Ashcroft, Oral History Interview, 2013.
7  Jean Golding, Oral History Interview, 2012.
8  Ethical considerations for the ALSPAC, draft memo by David Baum, November 1989 (ALSPAC Ethics Archive, A/89/11/24/1).
9  Jean Golding, Oral History Interview, 2012.
10  Ian Lister Cheese, Oral History Interview, 2013.
11  Hugh Barnes, personal correspondence, 7 April 2016.
12  Elizabeth Mumford, Oral History Interview, 2013.
13  Hugh Barnes, personal correspondence, 2 May 2013.
14  Tim Chambers, Oral History Interview, 2013.
15  Elizabeth Mumford, Oral History Interview, 2013.
16  Jean Golding, Oral History Interview, 2012.
17  Tim Chambers, Oral History Interview, 2013.

## Chapter Three: Advisory to independent: a missed opportunity

[1] See: http://webarchive.nationalarchives.gov.uk/20130107105354/ http://www.dh.gov.uk/prod_consum_dh/groups/dh_digitalassets/@dh/@en/documents/digitalasset/dh_4058609.pdf

[2] See: http://web.archive.org/web/20030423005717/http://www.alspac.bris.ac.uk/ALSPACext/MainProtocol/section3.htm

[3] Gordon Stirrat, Oral History Interview, 2013.

[4] Committee minutes, ALSPAC Ethics Archive, April 1994 to October 2000.

[5] See Figure 1: ALSPAC Management Structure, available at: http://web.archive.org/web/20030415152747/http://www.alspac.bris.ac.uk/ALSPACext/MainProtocol/Appendix1.htm

[6] Letter to Chair of District Medical and Ethical Committee from Jean Golding, 4 June 1990 (ALSPAC Ethics Archive, C/90/06/04/AM/JG/L).

[7] Committee minutes, ALSPAC Ethics Archive, November 2000 to July 2003.

[8] Committee minutes, ALSPAC Ethics Archive, from September 2003.

[9] Southmead REC:

Letter to Jean Golding from Secretary, 5 April 1990 (ALSPAC Ethics Archive, C/90/04/05/JG/ED/L)

Letter to Jean Golding from Secretary, 25 Aug 1992 (ALSPAC Ethics Archive, C/92/08/25/JG/SB/L/1)

Frenchay REC:

Letter to Jean Golding from Secretary, 25 July 1990 (ALSPAC Ethics Archive, C/90/07/25/JG/ERo/L)

Letter to Jean Golding from Secretary, 26 Nov 1992 (ALSPAC Ethics Archive, C/92/11/26/JG/PF/L)

Bristol & Weston REC:

Letter to Jean Golding from Chair, 10 Dec 1990 (ALSPAC Ethics Archive, C/90/12/10/JG/DS/L)

Letter to Jean Golding from Secretary, 4 June 1992 (ALSPAC Ethics Archive, C/92/06/04/JG/SH/L)

[10] See: www.hra.nhs.uk/resources/applying-to-recs/nhs-rec-directory/mergers-closures-rec-name-changes/

[11] Committee agenda, 10 August 1990 (ALSPAC Ethics Archive, A/90/08/10/A).

[12] Gordon Stirrat, Oral History Interview, 2013.

[13] Richard Ashcroft, Oral History Interview, 2013.

[14] Tim Chambers, Oral History Interview, 2013.

[15] Michael Furmston, Oral History Interview, 2012.

[16] Committee minutes, 17 November 1997 (ALSPAC Ethics Archive, A/97/11/17/M).

[17] See: http://web.archive.org/web/20030514055030/http://www.alspac.bris.ac.uk/ALSPACext/MainProtocol/COLLABORATION%20AND%20FUNDING.htm

[18] ALSPAC sub-studies (ALSPAC Ethics Archive, A/99/02/08/03).

[19] Committee minutes, 8 March 2004, Golombok, City University Ethics Committee approval (ALSPAC Ethics Archive, A/04/03/08/M).

[20] Committee minutes and memo to Committee, 16 October 1991 (ALSPAC Ethics Archive, A/91/10/16/M, A/91/10/16/2, A/91/11/09/M, A/91/12/02/M).

[21] See IRB00003312, available at: http://ohrp.cit.nih.gov/search/

[22] See Requirements for REC review, August 2011, available at: www.hra.nhs.uk/documents/2013/09/does-my-project-require-rec-review.pdf

## Chapter Four: Bureaucratic battles: liaison with the Local Research Ethics Committees

[1] Letter to Chair of LREC from David Baum, 11 August 1989 (ALSPAC Ethics Archive, C/89/08/11/XX/DB/L/1/3).

[2] Application for LREC approval (ALSPAC Ethics Archive, Appendix 1).

[3] LREC approval, 22 March 1991 (ALSPAC Ethics Archive, C/91/03/22/DST/SH/L).

[4] LREC approval, 8 October 1991 (ALSPAC Ethics Archive, C/91/10/08/JG/DS/L).

[5] Jean Golding, Oral History Interview, 2012.

[6] Update from Jean Golding to LRECs, 3 November 1993 (ALSPAC Ethics Archive, C/93/11/03/XX/JG/L).

[7] Letter to Jean Golding from LREC Chair, 6 June 1997 (ALSPAC Ethics Archive, C/97/08/06/JG/JA/L).

[8] LREC approval, 3 December 1997 (ALSPAC Ethics Archive, C/97/12/03/JG/NN/L).

[9] Letter to Jean Golding from LREC Secretary, 3 July 1997 (ALSPAC Ethics Archive, C/97/7/03/JG/SB/L).

[10] Tim Chambers, Oral History Interview, 2013.

[11] Committee minutes, 3 March 1998 (ALSPAC Ethics Archive, A/98/03/03/M).

[12] Letter to LREC Chair from Michael Furmston, 18 October 2004 (author's personal archive).

[13] Letter to Jean Golding from LREC Chair, 10th January 2005 (author's personal archive).

[14] Letter to LREC Chair from George Davey Smith, 8 January 2007 (author's personal archive).

[15] Memo: LREC problems for Shah Ebrahim, 2 February 2005 (author's personal archive).
[16] Letter to LREC Chair from Michael Furmston, 24 December 2004 (author's personal archive).
[17] Gordon Stirrat, Oral History Interview, 2013.
[18] Elizabeth Mumford, Oral History Interview, 2013.

## Chapter Five: Confidentiality and anonymity: a rod for their own backs

[1] See Figure 1 in Chapter One.
[2] ALSPAC Initial Participant Brochure (author's personal archive).
[3] Committee minutes, 3 August 1993 (ALSPAC Ethics Archive, A/93/08/03/M).
[4] Gordon Stirrat, Oral History Interview, 2013.
[5] ALSPAC data risk assessment: appendix 3i (author's personal archive).
[6] Committee minutes, 22 May 1991 (ALSPAC Ethics Archive, A/91/05/22/M).
[7] Committee minutes, 22 May 1991, 17 February 1993, 3 August 1993 (ALSPAC Ethics Archive, A/91/05/22/M, A/93/02/17/M, A/93/08/03/M).
[8] Committee minutes, 30 November 1990 (ALSPAC Ethics Archive, A/90/11/30/M).
[9] Committee minutes and Protocol for unsigned comments on questionnaires (ALSPAC Ethics Archive, A/04/01/19/M, A/04/01/19/7).
[10] Committee minutes, 3 September 2002 (ALSPAC Ethics Archive, A/02/09/03/M).
[11] Committee minutes, 15 April 1991 (ALSPAC Ethics Archive, A/91/04/15/M).
[12] Conditions for collaboration in ALSPAC, 19 July 1996 (ALSPAC Ethics Archive, A/96/07/19/2).
[13] Committee minutes, 28 February 2005, 21 March 2005, 11 April 2005, 5 May 2005, 31 May 2005, 4 July 2005 (ALSPAC Ethics Archive, A/05/02/28/M, A/05/03/21/M, A/05/04/11/M, A/05/05/05/M, A/05/05/31/M, A/05/07/04/M).

## Chapter Six: Informed consent: too much information

[1] Committee minutes, 22 May 1990 (ALSPAC Ethics Archive, A/90/05/22/M).
[2] ALSPAC Steering Committee minutes, 27 July 1989 (ALSPAC Administrative Archive, 1987–89).
[3] Committee minutes, 22 May 1990 (ALSPAC Ethics Archive, A/90/05/22/M).
[4] Committee minutes, 15 July 2003 (ALSPAC Ethics Archive, A/03/07/15/M).
[5] See: www.legislation.gov.uk/ukpga/1969/46
[6] Committee minutes, 22 May 1990 (ALSPAC Ethics Archive, A/90/05/22/M).

[7] Committee minutes and Bio-samples consent form, 22 May 1990, 29 October 1990 (ALSPAC Ethics Archive, A/90/05/22/M, A/90/10/29/M, A/90/10/29/1).

[8] Committee minutes, 28 October 1996 (ALSPAC Ethics Archive, A/96/10/28/M).

[9] Committee minutes, 2 July 1997 (ALSPAC Ethics Archive, A/97/07/02/M).

[10] Participant Information Sheet (genetics) (ALSPAC Ethics Archive, A/99/10/18/4/p).

[11] Committee minutes, 22 May 1990 (ALSPAC Ethics Archive, A/90/05/22/M).

[12] Committee minutes, 15 July 2003 (ALSPAC Ethics Archive, A/03/07/15/M).

[13] Committee minutes, 13 July 2000 (ALSPAC Ethics Archive, A/00/07/13/M).

[14] Committee minutes, 22 October 2002 (ALSPAC Ethics Archive, A/02/10/22/M).

[15] Committee minutes and Protocol for clinic consent by absent parents, 2 April 2001 (ALSPAC Ethics Archive, A/01/04/02/M, A/01/04/02/1).

[16] Committee minutes, 26 March 2002 (ALSPAC Ethics Archive, A/02/03/26/M).

[17] Committee minutes, 15 July 2003 (ALSPAC Ethics Archive, A/03/07/15/M).

## Chapter Seven: Child protection: an observational study?

[1] See: http://web.archive.org/web/20030309142314/http://www.alspac.bris. ac.uk/ALSPACext/MainProtocol/section2.htm

[2] Instructions for home interviewers, 22 August 1990 (ALSPAC Ethics Archive, A/09/08/22/1/b/i).

[3] Committee minutes, 22 August 1990 (ALSPAC Ethics Archive, A/90/08/22/M).

[4] Proposed hands-on assessments at age 7, 3 March 1998 (ALSPAC Ethics Archive, A/98/03/03/1).

[5] Committee minutes and ALSPAC Child Protection Policy, 10 December 2001 (ALSPAC Ethics Archive, A/01/12/10/M, A/01/12/10/2).

[6] Committee minutes, 15 September 2003 (ALSPAC Ethics Archive, A/03/09/15/M).

[7] Committee minutes and TF1 Psychosis Interview Child Protection Procedures, 26 September 2003 (ALSPAC Ethics Archive, A/03/09/26/M, A/03/09/26/2/c).

[8] Committee minutes, 5 May 2005 (ALSPAC Ethics Archive, A/05/05/05/M).

[9] Committee minutes, 15 September 2003 (ALSPAC Ethics Archive, A/03/09/15/M).

## Chapter Eight: Disclosure of individual results: foreseen feedback and incidental findings

[1] Committee minutes, 18 October 1999 (ALSPAC Ethics Archive, A/99/10/18/M).

[2] Notes on meeting of the Parents' Group Committee of ALSPAC, 8 May 1990 (author's personal archive).

[3] Committee minutes, 10 December 1990 (ALSPAC Ethics Archive, A/90/12/10/M).

[4] The provision of information to householders taking part in the Indoor Air Quality Study, 6 March 1991 (ALSPAC Ethics Archive, C/91/03/06/AEC/JG/A/1).

[5] Committee minutes, 14 January 1991 (ALSPAC Ethics Archive, A/91/01/14/M).

[6] Letter to collaborator from Jean Golding, 19 December 1994 (ALSPAC Ethics Archive, C/94/12/19/MS/JG).

[7] Committee minutes, 5 December 1994 (ALSPAC Ethics Archive, A/94/12/05/M).

[8] Committee minutes, 5 December 1994 (ALSPAC Ethics Archive, A/94/12/05/M).

[9] Committee minutes, 14 January 1991 (ALSPAC Ethics Archive, A/91/01/14/M).

[10] Committee minutes, 11 February 1991 (ALSPAC Ethics Archive, A/91/02/11/M).

[11] Committee minutes and Ultrasound scan interviews preliminary results, 8 March 1991, 15 April 1991 (ALSPAC Ethics Archive, A/91/03/08/M, A/91/04/15/M, A/91/04/15/1).

[12] Committee minutes, 24 September 1991 (ALSPAC Ethics Archive, A/91/09/24/M).

[13] Committee minutes, 2 December 1991 (ALSPAC Ethics Archive, A/91/12/02/M).

[14] See: www.bristol.ac.uk/alspac/

[15] Committee minutes, 2 December 1991 (ALSPAC Ethics Archive, A/91/12/02/M).

[16] Screening for plasma total cholesterol and Committee minutes, 26 April 1994, 6 February 1995 (ALSPAC Ethics Archive, A/94/04/26/1/p/a, A/95/02/06/M).

[17] Personal communication from Jean Golding.

[18] Draft Participant Information Sheet: the 10%Club, 12 August 1992 (ALSPAC Ethics Archive, A/92/08/12/1/p).

[19] Letter to Jean Golding from collaborator, 23 April 1998 (ALSPAC Ethics Archive, C/98/04/23/JG/PW).

[20] Committee minutes, 3 March 1998 (ALSPAC Ethics Archive, A/98/03/03/M).

[21] Committee minutes, 8 December 1992 (ALSPAC Ethics Archive, A/92/12/08/M).

[22] Memo to Jean Golding from Sue Sadler, Clinic Manager, 10 December 1995 (author's personal archive)

[23] Letters to parents and GPs disclosing results, 30 September 1997 (ALSPAC Ethics Archive, A/97/09/30/7).

[24] Letter to parents re abnormal hearing (ALSPAC Ethics Archive, A/98/07/22/8/a).

[25] F@7 referral letter hearing deficiency (author's personal archive).

[26] Letter to collaborator from Jean Golding, 19 December 1994 (ALSPAC Ethics Archive, C/94/12/19/MS/JG).

[27] Committee minutes, 6 September 2004 (ALSPAC Ethics Archive, A/04/09/06/M).

[28] Committee minutes, 20 September 2004 (ALSPAC Ethics Archive, A/04/09/20/M).

[29] Committee minutes, 6 September 2004 (ALSPAC Ethics Archive, A/04/09/06/M).

[30] UK Biobank participant leaflet, available at: www.ukbiobank.ac.uk/wp-content/uploads/2011/06/Participant_information_leaflet.pdf?phpMyAdmin=trmKQlYdjjnQlgJ%2CfAzikMhEnx6

[31] ALSPAC Disclosure of Results Policy, available at: www.bristol.ac.uk/media-library/sites/alspac/migrated/documents/alspac-disclosure-policy.pdf

## Chapter Nine: Disclosure of individual results: participants' requests

[1] Personal correspondence, author to Elizabeth Mumford, 14 July 2006.

[2] Committee minutes, 12 March 2001 (ALSPAC Ethics Archive, A/01/03/12/M).

## Chapter Ten: Participants' problems: people not policies

[1] ALSPAC Initial Participant Brochure (author's personal archive).

[2] Committee minutes, 17 February 1992 (ALSPAC Ethics Archive, A/92/02/17/M).

[3] Committee minutes, 5 December 1994 (ALSPAC Ethics Archive, A/94/12/05/M).

[4] Committee minutes, 1 May 1995 (ALSPAC Ethics Archive, A/95/05/01/M).

[5] Committee minutes, 30 September 1997 (ALSPAC Ethics Archive, A/97/09/30/M).

[6] Committee minutes, 17 November 1997 (ALSPAC Ethics Archive, A/97/11/17/M).

[7] Committee minutes, 22 May 1991 (ALSPAC Ethics Archive, A/91/05/22/M).

[8] Incident report, 2 April 1996 (ALSPAC Ethics Archive, A/96/05/13/1/d).

[9] Committee minutes, 13 May 1996 (ALSPAC Ethics Archive, A/96/05/13/M).

[10] Committee minutes, 19 November 2002 (ALSPAC Ethics Archive, A/02/11/19/M).

[11] Committee minutes and Letter to participants concerning miscarriage, 8 October 1990, 29 October 1990 (ALSPAC Ethics Archive, A/90/10/08/M, A/90/10/29/M, A/90/10/29/2).

[12] Committee minutes, 15 April 1991 (ALSPAC Ethics Archive, A/91/04/15/M).

[13] Committee minutes, 22 May 1991 (ALSPAC Ethics Archive, A/91/05/22/M).

[14] Committee minutes, 12 February 2001 (ALSPAC Ethics Archive, A/01/02/12/M).

## Chapter Eleven: External databases: anonymous linkage

[1] Initial Ethics Application to Bristol and Weston LREC (ALSPAC Ethics Archive, Appendix 1, Initial Application).

[2] Committee minutes, 11 April 2005 (ALSPAC Ethics Archive, A/05/04/11/M).

[3] Committee minutes and Teacher and Head Teacher Questionnaires, 29 June 1999, 22 July 1999 (ALSPAC Ethics Archive, A/99/06/29/M, A/99/06/29/2/a-c, A/99/07/22/M).

[4] Committee minutes, 6 November 2001 (ALSPAC Ethics Archive, A/01/11/06/M).

[5] Committee minutes, 23 July 2002 (ALSPAC Ethics Archive, A/02/07/23/M).

[6] Committee minutes, 3 March 2003 (ALSPAC Ethics Archive, A/03/03/03/M).

[7] Committee minutes, 21 May 2003 (ALSPAC Ethics Archive, A/03/05/21/M).

[8] Committee minutes and newsletter articles, 17 June 2003 (ALSPAC Ethics Archive, A/03/06/17/M, A/03/06/17/6-7).

[9] Committee minutes, 26 September 2003 (ALSPAC Ethics Archive, A/03/09/26/M).

## Chapter Twelve: Retention of the cohort: incentives or inducements

[1] Committee minutes, 13 November 2003 (ALSPAC Ethics Archive, A/03/11/13/M).

[2] Committee minutes and newsletter article, 9 May 2000 (ALSPAC Ethics Archive, A/00/05/09/M, A/00/05/09/1/b).

3   Committee minutes, 7 September 2000 (ALSPAC Ethics Archive, A/00/09/07/M).
4   Committee minutes, 17 May 2004 (ALSPAC Ethics Archive, A/04/05/17/M).

## Chapter Thirteen: Commercial collaborations: selling our souls

1   Committee minutes, 6 February 1995 (ALSPAC Ethics Archive, A/95/02/06/M).
2   ALSPAC participants' newsletter No 17.
3   Personal correspondence from Jean Golding.
4   Committee minutes, 7 September 2000 (ALSPAC Ethics Archive, A/00/09/07/M).
5   Jean Golding, personal archive.
6   Committee minutes, 7 September 2000 (ALSPAC Ethics Archive, A/00/09/07/M).
7   Committee minutes, 13 July 2000 (ALSPAC Ethics Archive, A/00/07/13/M).
8   Committee minutes, 2 May 2001 (ALSPAC Ethics Archive, A/01/05/02/M).
9   Committee minutes, 18 December 2000, 11 January 2001, 12 March 2001, 2 May 2001 (ALSPAC Ethics Archive, A/00/12/18/M, A/01/01/11/M, A/01/03/12/M, A/01/05/02/M).
10  Committee minutes, 2 May 2001 (ALSPAC Ethics Archive, A/01/05/02/M/p).
11  Committee minutes, 10 October 2001 (ALSPAC Ethics Archive, A/01/10/10/M).
12  Genetics Knowledge Park abstract, 6 November 2001 (ALSPAC Ethics Archive, A/01/11/06/1).
13  Committee minutes, 6 November 2001 (ALSPAC Ethics Archive, A/01/11/06/M).
14  Committee minutes, 10 December 2001 (ALSPAC Ethics Archive, A/01/12/10/M).
15  Committee minutes, 26 March 2002 (ALSPAC Ethics Archive, A/02/03/26/M).
16  Committee minutes, 26 March 2002 (ALSPAC Ethics Archive, A/02/03/26/M)
17  Committee minutes, 29 April 2003 (ALSPAC Ethics Archive, A/03/04/29/M).
18  Committee minutes, 15 July 2003 (ALSPAC Ethics Archive, A/03/07/15/M).
19  Committee minutes, 17 May 2004 (ALSPAC Ethics Archive, A/04/05/17/M).
20  Committee minutes, 29 April 2003 (ALSPAC Ethics Archive, A/03/04/29/M).
21  Committee minutes, 15 July 2003 (ALSPAC Ethics Archive, A/03/07/15/M).

## Chapter Fourteen: Comprehensive oversight: undocumented and unacknowledged

[1] David Jewell, Oral History Interview, 2012.

[2] Committee minutes, 13 November 2003 (ALSPAC Ethics Archive, A/03/11/13/M).

[3] David Jewell, Oral History Interview, 2012.

[4] Committee minutes, 4 December 1998 (ALSPAC Ethics Archive, A/98/12/04/M).

[5] Committee minutes, 5 July 1990 (ALSPAC Ethics Archive, A/90/07/05/M).

[6] Committee minutes, 2 January 2003 (ALSPAC Ethics Archive, A/03/01/02/M).

[7] ALSPAC Children in Focus; blood taking methodology, available at: http://web.archive.org/web/20030501234603/http://www.alspac.bris.ac.uk/ALSPACext/MainProtocol/Appendix7/Child_Focus7.htm#blood_taking

[8] ALSPAC Aims and Study Design: Appendix 1: the ALSPAC advisory and management structures, available at: http://web.archive.org/web/20030415152747/http://www.alspac.bris.ac.uk/ALSPACext/MainProtocol/Appendix1.htm

[9] Update of sub-studies, 8 February 1999 (ALSPAC Ethics Archive, A/99/02/08/3).

## Chapter Fifteen: Influence beyond ALSPAC: extension of expertise

[1] Marcus Pembrey, Oral History Interview, 2013.

[2] See: www.nature.com/ejhg/journal/v11/n2s/index.html

[3] Letter to Michael Furmston from Marcus Pembrey, 23 June 1999 (ALSPAC Ethics Archive, C/99/06/23/MF/MP).

[4] Call for evidence: Inquiry into Human Genetic Databases, 20 July 2000 (ALSPAC Ethics Archive, A/00/08/02/6).

[5] Committee minutes, 18 December 2000 (ALSPAC Ethics Archive, A/00/12/18/M).

[6] Inquiry into Human Genetic Databases (House of Lords Science and Technology Sub-Committee) draft response, 11 October 2000 (ALSPAC Ethics Archive, A/00/10/11/1).

[7] See: www.publications.parliament.uk/pa/ld200809/ldselect/ldsctech/107/107we33.htm

[8] Committee minutes, 10 February 2004 (ALSPAC Ethics Archive, A/04/02/10/M).

[9] Draft presentations for Human Genetics Commission, 12 May 2004 (author's personal archive).

[10] Committee minutes, 17 May 2004 (ALSPAC Ethics Archive, A/04/05/17/M).

[11] See: www.ukbiobank.ac.uk/ethics/

[12] Committee minutes, 18 October 2004 (ALSPAC Ethics Archive, A/04/10/18/M).

[13] Committee minutes, 11 April 2005 (ALSPAC Ethics Archive, A/05/04/11/M).

[14] In May 1999, Marcus Pembrey attended a Wellcome Trust workshop to discuss plans for a UK Population Biomedical Collection (later to become UK Biobank).

[15] See: www.publications.parliament.uk/pa/ld200809/ldselect/ldsctech/107/8101509.htm

[16] Committee minutes, 15 July 2003 (ALSPAC Ethics Archive, A/03/07/15/M).

## Conclusions

[1] Jean Golding, Oral History Interview, 2012.

[2] www.bristol.ac.uk/golding/ (accessed February 2017).

[3] ALSPAC Initial Participant Brochure (author's personal archive).

[4] Tim Chambers, Oral History Interview, 2013.

[5] Draft application for Wellcome Trust biomedical ethics research grant, 8 February 1999 (ALSPAC Ethics Archive, A/99/02/08/2).

[6] Ethical Protection in Epidemiological Genetic Research: Participants' Perspectives, available at: www.bris.ac.uk/Depts//Ethics/CEM/epeg_background.htm

[7] Richard Ashcroft, Oral History Interview, 2013.

# References

Al-Shahi, R. (2005) 'Research ethics committees in the UK – the pressure is now on research and development departments', *Journal of the Royal Society of Medicine*, vol 98, no 10, pp 444–7.

Birmingham, K. and Doyle, A. (2009) 'Ethics and governance of a longitudinal birth cohort', *Paediatric & Perinatal Epidemiology*, vol 23, suppl 1, pp 39–50.

BPA (British Paediatric Association Ethics Advisory Committee) (1992) *Guidelines for the ethical conduct of medical research involving children*, London: British Paediatric Association.

Caulfield, T., Upshur, R. and Daar, A. (2003) 'DNA databanks and consent: a suggested policy option involving an authorization model', *BMC Medical Ethics*, vol 4, no 1, p 1.

CIOMS (Council for International Organizations of Medical Sciences) (1991) 'World Health Organization', International Guidelines for Ethical Review of Epidemiological Studies, Geneva.

Fraser, A., Macdonald-Wallis, C., Tilling, K., Boyd, A., Golding, J., Davey Smith, G., Henderson, J., Macleod, J., Molloy, L., Ness, A., Ring, S., Nelson, S.M. and Lawlor, D.A. (2012) 'Cohort profile: the Avon Longitudinal Study of Parents and Children: ALSPAC mothers' cohort', *International Journal of Epidemiology*, vol 42, no 1, pp 97–110.

Glasziou, P. and Chalmers, I. (2004) 'Ethics review roulette: what can we learn?', *British Medical Journal*, vol 328, pp 121–2.

Godard, B., Schmidtke, J., Cassiman, J. and Aymé, S. (2003) 'Data storage and DNA banking for biomedical research: informed consent, confidentiality, quality issues, ownership, return of benefits. A professional perspective', *European Journal of Human Genetics*, vol 11, suppl 2, pp 88–122.

Golding, J. (1989a) 'European Longitudinal Study of Pregnancy and Childhood (ELSPAC)', *Paediatric and Perinatal Epidemiology*, vol 3, no 4, pp 460–9.

Golding, J. (1989b) 'Study on factors influencing child health', *The Lancet*, vol 334 (originally vol 2), no 8661, p 518.

Golding, J., Greenwood, R., Birmingham, K. and Mott, M. (1992) 'Childhood cancer, intramuscular vitamin K, and pethidine given during labour', *British Medical Journal*, vol 305, no 6849, pp 341–6.

Golding, J., Birmingham, K.E. and Jones, R.W. (eds) (2009) 'A guide to undertaking a birth cohort study: purposes, pitfalls and practicalities', *Paediatric and Perinatal Epidemiology*, vol 23, suppl 1.

Jones, R., Pembrey, M., Golding, J. and Herrick, D. (2005) 'The search for genenotype/phenotype associations and the phenome scan', *Paediatric and Perinatal Epidemiology*, vol 19, no 4, pp 264–75.

Kent, J., Williamson, E., Goodenough, T. and Ashcroft, R. (2002) 'Social science gets the ethics treatment: research governance and ethical review', *Sociological Research Online*, vol 7, no 4, www.socresonline.org.uk/7/4/williamson.html.

Lowrance, W. (2002) *Learning from experience: Privacy and the secondary use of data in health research*, London: Nuffield Trust.

Metcalfe, C., Martin, R.M. and Noble, S. (2008) 'Low risk research using routinely collected identifiable health information without informed consent: encounters with the Patient Information Advisory Group', *Journal of Medical Ethics*, vol 34, no 1, pp 37–40.

MRC (Medical Research Council) (1991) *The ethical conduct of research on children*, London: MRC.

MRC (2005) *Medical Research Council position statement on research regulation and ethics*, London: MRC.

Mumford, S.E. (1999a) 'Children of the 90s: ethical guidance for a longitudinal study', *Archives of Disease in Childhood. Fetal and Neonatal Edition*, vol 81, no 2, pp 146–51.

Mumford, S.E. (1999b) 'Children of the 90s II: challenges for the ethics and law committee', *Archives of Disease in Childhood. Fetal and Neonatal Edition*, vol 81, no 3, pp 228–31.

O'Hare, D. (2014) 'Working with policy makers and the public in ALSPAC', *Society for Longitudinal and Life Course Studies International Journal*, vol 6, no 1, p 2.

O'Neill, O. (2003) 'Some limits of informed consent', *Journal of Medical Ethics*, vol 29, pp 4–7.

Overy, C., Reynolds, L.A. and Tansey, E.M. (eds) (2012) *History of the Avon Longitudinal Study of Parents & Children (ALSPAC) c. 1980–2000, Wellcome witnesses to 20th century medicine* (vol 44), London: Queen Mary, University of London.

RCP (Royal College of Physicians) (1990) 'Research involving patients: summary and recommendations of a report of the Royal College of Physicians', *Journal of the Royal College of Physicians of London*, vol 24, no 1, pp 10–14.

World Medical Association (1964) 'Declaration of Helsinki' (revised 1975, 1982, 1989).

# Appendix 1:
# ALSPAC Steering Committee:
# founding members

From ALSPAC Steering Committee minutes, 1987–89, page 164
(ALSPAC Administrative Archive)

- Dr Jean Golding (Chair), Institute of Child Health, Bristol
- Professor Catherine Peckham, Institute of Child Health, London
- Professor Marcus Pembrey, Institute of Child Health, London
- Professor David Baum, Institute of Child Health, Bristol
- Professor Gordon Stirrat, Department of Obstetrics & Gynaecology, University of Bristol
- Dr Charles Pennock, Department of Pathology and Child Health, University of Bristol
- Dr Jon Pollock (Secretary), Institute of Child Health, Bristol

# Appendix 2:
# ALSPAC Ethics and Law Committee members: appointed 1990–2005

| | | |
|---|---|---|
| Ashcroft, Richard | Ethicist | 09/09/1998 to 31/03/2000 |
| Bailey, Sarah | Study Mother | 08/02/1999 to 23/05/2002 |
| Barnes, Hugh | Child Psychiatrist | 13/06/2000 to 31/03/2014 |
| Baum, David | Professor of Child Health | 25/04/1990 to 24/03/1997 |
| Bertram, Chris | Philosopher | 07/09/2000 to 17/10/2005 |
| Karen Birmingham | Research Nurse | 01/12/1999 to 31/03/2014 Secretary throughout |
| Bowles, Ruth | Study Mother | 12/03/2001 to present |
| Bryer, Sheila | Study Mother | 05/12/1994 to 05/07/1996 |
| Cadman, Marilyn | Study Mother | 08/02/1999 to 18/12/2000 |
| Campbell, Alastair | Professor of Ethics in Medicine | 28/10/1996 to 03/03/1998 |
| Chambers, Tim | Consultant Paediatrician | 22/05/1990 to 02/06/1997 |
| Furmston, Michael | Professor of Law | 25/04/1990 to 19/02/2008 Chair 25/04/1990 to 05/09/2006 |
| Golding, Jean | Director of ALSPAC | 25/04/1990 to 02/01/2009 |
| Henderson, John | Paediatrician | 08/05/1997 to 17/10/2005 |
| Hirschmann, David | Philosopher | 25/04/1990 to 24/03/1997 |
| Jewell, David | General Practitioner | 13/06/2000 to 03/09/2013 Chair 09/03/2010 to 03/09/2013 |

| Keen, Peter | Dean of the Faculty of Medicine | 25/04/1990 to 12/12/1995 |
|---|---|---|
| King, Ursula | Professor of Theology | 25/04/1990 to 10/12/1991 |
| Lister Cheese, Ian | Senior Medical Officer, Department of Health | 25/04/1990 to 12/12/1995 Re-joined 19/07/1996 to 18/07/2000 |
| Mumford, Elizabeth née Roberts | Lawyer, Expert on Medical Law | 25/04/1990 to 06/10/2011 Secretary 25/04/1990 to 18/10/1999 |
| Ness, Andy | Epidemiologist | 29/04/2003 to 17/10/2005 |
| Nott, Jan | School Nurse | 30/09/2002 to 07/08/2008 |
| O'Day, Ken | Philosopher | 03/11/1997 to 29/05/2000 |
| Scholar, Phillippa | Teacher | 11/10/2004 to 05/09/2006 |
| Stirrat, Gordon | Obstetrician | 25/04/1990 to 09/05/2000 Re-joined 23/05/2002 to 15/12/2009 Chair 20/09/2006 to 15/12/2009 |
| Wallace, Ruth | Study Mother | 03/09/2002 to 09/03/2010 |
| Watson, Norma | Head teacher of Primary School | 13/07/2000 to 06/09/2004 |
| Webster Green, Joanna | Study Mother | 08/05/1997 to 19/01/1998 |
| Williamson, Chris | Health Visitor | 05/02/1996 to 03/09/2002 |

# Appendix 3:
# Letter to participants: further information concerning confidentiality

# The Avon Longitudinal Study of Pregnancy and Childhood
## (ALSPAC)

**Children of the Nineties**
University of Bristol
24 Tyndall Avenue
Bristol, BS2 8BJ

Tel: (0272) 256260
Fax: (0272) 255051

Dear

Date:

We appreciate your concern about the Children of the Nineties data, but hope that the following notes will remove any worries that you might have. The need to ensure the privacy and confidentiality of the data about you and your child has been a central part of the study design from the beginning. The local NHS ethics committees have discussed and approved the study, and we have registered its existence with the Data Protection Registrar, to comply with the 1984 Data Protection Act. Both the ethics committees and the Data Protection Act state principles which we abide by, and they serve to protect you and your rights.

## Data collection

We do hope that you will support the study as much as you can, as that will greatly increase its success, but of course your co-operation at any stage is voluntary. You can ignore any sections of the questionnaires we send you, and if you say you do not want to help at all, we will respect your wishes. The blood, urine and placenta samples will be passed to us by the hospital laboratory staff only if there is some spare after being used for the normal monitoring and maintenance of the health of you and your baby. We will analyse these samples only with your consent.

## The computer systems

We shall be using two separate computers in this study, one to store personal identifiers and the other for survey results.

## 1. Personal identifiers.

To run the survey, we need to know your name, address and estimated date of delivery. If you change your address, we would like you to tell us. We note such items as the sex and date of birth of your baby. All that data is put into a computer, so that we can print address labels for your questionnaires, and so that we can send them to you at fixed stages in your pregnancy and in the early life of your child. These items are completely confidential, but we do need them to be able to contact you about the questionnaires, and to send you information about the survey. Should you tell us that you do not want to continue with the survey, then your computer entry is changed so that you hear no more from us.

Each questionnaire has a code number on it, and we keep a note on the first computer of who has been sent which code number. When you return the questionnaire, we use that number to check it back in. After a while, we send out reminders to those people whose questionnaires have not come back yet.

The contact number which we send to you at the start of the survey is only for you to use if you phone up with a query. It

Steering Committee:
*Professor J. D. Baum, Professor G. M. Stirrat,*
*Professor M. Pembrey, Professor C. Peckham, Dr. J. Golding,*
*Professor M. Rutter, Dr. C. Pennock, Dr. J. I. Pollock.*

is also stored on the first computer, and enables us to call up your entry easily, if it needs to be corrected, or you've lost your questionnaire, or whatever.

## 2. Survey responses.

The answers you give on the questionnaires are not put into the same computer as that which has your name and address. They are put into a second machine, run by a different set of people, and it does not have your name and address in it at all. This means that there is no link in any one computer between who you are, and how you have answered the questions. The people analysing the questionnaires will <u>not</u> know, and will not need to know, who filled them in. If you phone the hotline with your contact number, the person who speaks to you will <u>not</u> be able to read your answers to the questions. The results of blood, urine and cell sample analyses are dealt with in the same sort of way. They are not associated in any one computer with your name and address.

## What if the computers get it wrong?

Your GP and hospital look after you and your baby in the normal way. No data that we collect about you is used to control or change your treatment. Indeed, the study design which separates your name and address from your other data stops us from doing that. So if there are mistakes on our computers, it cannot affect you. Nevertheless it is important to us that the data is as accurate as possible, and there are many checks in the computers to maintain this accuracy. You may spot some errors – maybe for example we will get your baby's date of birth down incorrectly – please let us know if you notice any mistakes.

The data is only used for the purposes of the survey, and is not passed on for other use.

Because the data are collected only for statistical research purposes, we are exempt from providing access to their own data to individual study participants. (1984 Data Protection Act sect 33 para 6).

## Security.

We use two secure computing systems to hold the data, and the returned questionnaires are destroyed after they have been keyed and validated. Staff working on the project are selected for discretion, and have signed undertakings to maintain absolute confidentiality about all material collected.

We appreciate your concern about the study. It is not possible to describe the system in any greater detail to you without beginning to compromise the security of the whole survey. These notes show you how we have taken the need to protect the individual to the heart of the study design. Thank you for your interest, and we do hope that you will continue to be part of "Children of the Nineties".

Yours sincerely,

Hugh Simmons, Manager : Children of the Nineties

# Appendix 4:
# Young Mothers paper by
# Elizabeth Mumford

ALSPAC Young Mothers

Although I was asked specifically to look at the question of young mothers (i.e. those under 16 or 18), it seems to me that there are similar problems when adult mothers are incompetent (through physical or mental illness or handicap).

I Young Mothers

A) Mothers Under 16: Unlawful Sexual Intercourse

Under the Sexual Offences Act 1956, it is an offence for a man to have sexual intercourse with a girl under the age of 16. Thus, if a girl is pregnant at 16, her partner will inevitably have committed an offence. It is not, however, an offence for the girl herself to have under-age sexual relations, nor can she be guilty of aiding and abetting the boy/man, as she is perceived to be the victim of the offence.

From the point of view of the study, it would seem important that there be no way of identifying the partner of a mother who was under 16 at the time of conception. If we do not know his identity, we can assure the girl that the matter will be kept confidential. We can also avoid being subpoenaed (although this would be unlikely) in any prosecution of the partner for the above-mentioned offences.

There is, of course, the possibility that the girl's pregnancy is the result of incest or other sexual abuse. This might become evident in the course of an interview, in which case, we would be faced with the usual dilemma about what to disclose and to whom. There is also the separate question about whether the fact of a close genetic relationship between mother and father would be something about which those working on the genetic material should know.

B) Consent

1) To the taking of biological samples

The Family Law Reform Act 1969 states at s.8 that minors who have reached the age of 16 are competent to give valid consent to "medical treatment" etc. As the primary purpose for which the sample is being taken is to assess maternal/foetal health, this would seem to fit within the section and render the consent of a mother over 16 valid to the actual insertion of the needle and drawing of blood.

As regards mothers under 16, the law was clarified by the Gillick decision in the House of Lords. Nothing in statute or common law prohibits such children from giving consent to treatment and the test of whether an individual is competent to do so becomes one of her understanding and maturity, couple with the doctor's view that the procedure in question is in her interests. Thus, most of our young mothers would have the right to consent to the withdrawal of blood for testing.

There is however some question as to whether a young woman is entitled in law to allow her blood to be further used for research purposes. Contracts purported to be entered into by minors are not usually legally binding, nor are minors entitled to dispose of their property by gift or sale unless it is to their benefit. While it is clear that the consent form we use is not a contract, there is some question as to whether the person who provides blood or tissue has some property interest in it. The answer is far from clear, as the case law in the past has dealt more with money and tangible property. The most likely interpretation, in my view, is that the transaction would be seen as being "voidable" – that is to say that the girl could change her mind on reaching majority and choose to withdraw from the study and to have her samples destroyed – which of course she could do in any case. Incidentally, the answer is not to ask for permission from the girl's parents, for they do not have the power to dispose of their minor children's property either.

Using a different analogy – that of harm to the person rather than harm to some alleged property interest – it is possible under certain circumstances for a mature and comprehending minor to consent to things which are not for his or her benefit and which may be positively harmful. The mere fact that Parliament has had to enact statutes such as the Tattooing of Minors Act and the provisions on under-age sex suggests that in the absence of specific legislation, the minor's consent is valid.

Finally, it is hard to think of what action might be brought against ALSPAC in this regard, as long as we have ensured that the girl in question is fully aware of what is intended in the use and storage of biological material and has consented.

2) The Questionnaires and Interviews

In general, it is probably the case that one is entitled to ask anyone anything one likes, whether the subject is a child or an adult. There are, however, one or two problems with these particular questions. The first is the practical matter of sending questionnaires to a home where it is possible that some or all family members are unaware of the girl's pregnancy, or where the girl has not yet accepted the fact that she is pregnant or decided whether or not to keep the baby (both situations are quite prevalent among young mothers).

From the legal point of view, there are two additional issues. The first concerns the rather old-fashioned idea that it is for the parent to decide the place and manner in which the child spends her time. (Children Act 1975—This phrase, but not, I think, the concept- will disappear with the coming into force of the Children Act 1989 next year). Presumably control of the girl's time includes whether or not she is to be filling in questionnaires or talking for two hours to an interviewer. Added to this is the fact that the interviewer may well be calling to see the teen-aged mother at her parents' home: thus, presumably they have some right to determine who will be received there and to insist on remaining present during the interview if they wish.

My feeling is that it is probably best to wait for complaints, rather than actively to seek parental consent to the girl's participation, but I am not sure I have the right answer here.

The other matter is that of the questions on sexual history. There is a fine line between legitimate activities such as sex education (and, I think, this study) and activities which, when the subject is a minor, might be construed as the common law offence of outraging public decency (I am thinking here of a recent case actually involving a home-made "questionnaire" about sexual activities which a schoolmaster had two boys read aloud to him and as a result of which he was charged). It might be prudent to omit the sex questions where the mother is under 16.

C) Mothers who are wards of course or in local authority care

I am not an expert in this area, but my feeling is that there is no substantial different between the position of these and other minor girls, as parent substitutes are required to act, at least for these purposes, exactly as parents would and thus have the same responsibilities.

II. Incompetent Mothers.

This category includes the cases of very young mothers who do not have the maturity to give consent or to answer questions and mothers, whether minors or not, who lack capacity due to mental handicap or mental or physical illness.

Presumably, it would still be of interest to have information about such women and this might be provided by their parents, guardians or other family members. The decision about whether a woman was capable of participating would ideally be made by the midwife/G.P. and following this, the questionnaires might be altered so as to eliminate those things which could not be answered by proxy (e.g. state of mind).

As concerns the biological material, it seems to be clear law that the parent of a minor may consent to his or her child's participation in medical procedures that are not necessary to the child's health (there are cases on blood testing for paternity) as long it is a "reasonable" decision for a parent to make and is not manifestly against the child's interests. This would presumably apply here and <u>might </u>be extended to include adult incompetents. The question of property is again a difficult one. However, it is possible that an adult incompetent will have a guardian under the Mental Health Act, appointed to deal with her property. In such a case that person (if not the parent) it might be wise also to ask his/her consent to the biological testing.

\*\*\*\*\*

It might also be of interest at some point to discuss the question of women who are intending unusual parenting arrangements (surrogacy, ovum donation or even adoption). These cases may present both administrative and technical challenges.

E. Books.

# Appendix 5:
# The Children of the Nineties study (ALSPAC) and collaboration with pharmaceutical companies

The 'Children of the Nineties' study (ALSPAC) is dedicated to understanding the environmental and genetic influences on development from infancy to adult life, and how these affect our health and well-being. Eventually, the study will suggest ways in which common diseases in childhood and adult life can be prevented, or treated.

## Principles underlying research in ALSPAC

A fundamental principle that governs the conduct of ALSPAC is that, like most studies supported by public agencies and charities, the discoveries that are made will end up in the public domain. There, they can be accessed freely by the international research community, by those who shape and provide public health services, by commercial companies searching for and developing new medicines, and, indeed, by any person or agency with an interest in health and welfare. ALSPAC recognises that the willingness of cohort families to continue giving so much of their time to the project depends on the protection of the principle that discoveries that come from the project are ultimately for the benefit of all.

## Support for research in ALSPAC

Bristol University, the Medical Research Council, the Wellcome Trust and other organisations provide ALSPAC with funds that help to maintain many of its 'core' functions, for example, the organisation of clinics, computer programming, statistics and communication with cohort members. However, this 'core' funding does not cover the exploitation of the research opportunities provided by the study. Consequently, ALSPAC and its collaborators must still seek funding for much of the collection, measurement and analysis of information from the cohort. Raising money to support research in ALSPAC is a major task for both ALSPAC and its collaborators, and success in doing so is critical in ensuring the study's continued productivity.

Proposals for scientific work utilising the ALSPAC resource are initially scrutinised by ALSPAC's advisory committees. The Law and Ethics Committee decides whether a project meets the required ethical standards, and other committees advise on whether a project reaches the necessary scientific standard. Subsequently, the fully costed proposal is submitted to grant-giving organisations (government research councils, or various charitable organisations), where they are subject to further independent review.

If a project meets the required (high) standard and is financially supported, arrangements are made to provide the research group, which may be based anywhere in the UK, or further afield, with access to the information and samples in ALSPAC that they need in order to answer their scientific question. If DNA samples need to be analysed as part of the project, small amounts of DNA from all the samples in the ALSPAC DNA bank are sent to a laboratory for the necessary measurements. The samples are completely anonymous as far as that laboratory is concerned. When the genetic analysis has been carried out, the results are returned to ALSPAC and linked with other information about the individuals whose DNA has been analysed. It is this process that allows statisticians to establish, for example, whether any genetic variation among cohort members is associated with a particular outcome or test result, for example, with being tall, or being more likely to suffer from eczema, or with being fat and so on.

The value of ALSPAC is in the research that makes sense of all the information and samples, including DNA, which are held by it. Without research, the information and samples by themselves are of little or no value. ALSPAC does not 'sell' its resources, but shares them with the scientific community and, as a consequence, adds to the sum total of knowledge in the public domain by publishing the results in scientific journals and by disseminating information more widely through the press. The whole research process is controlled so that all the interests of ALSPAC and the cohort's members (children and parents) are met.

## Benefiting from the results of ALSPAC's research

Pharmaceutical companies are among the many organisations that will benefit from the advances being made in understanding human genetic make-up. Information about what our genes do and how their functions contribute to a complete human being can provide clues to the design of new drugs. For example, by knowing all the genes that are responsible for the components of our immune systems, we can identify these components as possible targets for drugs that could be used to treat allergies, viral infections or autoimmune diseases. However, much of this part of drug discovery takes place in laboratories where the systems used to search for useful drugs are very simple when compared with a complete person living their life in a complex environment. Consequently, there is a large gap between discovering a possible drug and showing that it will have a beneficial effect and, importantly, be free of damaging side effects.

Part of the research that ALSPAC supports aims to discover how our individual genetic make-up affects the likelihood that we will develop common diseases, such as asthma, heart disease or adult diabetes. If we discovered that a particular version of a gene makes us more susceptible to asthma, then this would demonstrate that the product of this gene makes a critical contribution to the development of the disease. This in turn makes this product a good candidate as a target for drugs designed to protect against or treat asthma. Equally (or more) importantly, because so much information is collected about each individual in ALSPAC, it is possible to discover whether changes in the properties of a gene have other effects on our health. This provides important clues as to whether a drug aimed at the gene product could have significant side effects and therefore be unsafe.

## Adding value to ALSPAC

The results of research carried out in ALSPAC will contain information valuable to the pharmaceutical industry, which they will be able to access freely, along with everyone else, when it enters the public domain. Given ALSPAC's need for financial support for research projects, there is a strong argument for inviting pharmaceutical companies to provide direct support for those projects where the results will be valuable to them. Indeed, important funders of ALSPAC, such as the Medical Research Council and the Wellcome Trust, expect that this will happen.

The conditions under which pharmaceutical firms would undertake collaborative research in ALSPAC would be at least as stringent as those that apply to academic collaborators. Indeed, commercial companies would expect that the conditions of collaboration would be legally binding. There would be no 'sale' of DNA or information, confidentiality would be protected, there would be a period during which the results would remain confidential to ALSPAC and the collaborating company, and the results would finally be published so they entered the public domain. The pharmaceutical company would learn more about the potential effectiveness and safety of its drugs.

ALSPAC would gain support for its research activities and add to the total sum of information produced by the study, which would not only contribute to the development of new drugs, but also further our understanding of the development of disease and might point to other forms of prevention or treatment.

## Conclusion

ALSPAC must continue to seek support for the research that will give value to the wealth of information that it has collected over the last 10 years and that it continues to collect. The results of this research will be valuable to many, including the pharmaceutical industry, and it makes sense to seek support from them for the research from which they and everyone else will ultimately benefit. Provided this is done on the basis of agreements that do not compromise the overall aims of ALSPAC, or its relationship with the children and parents on whose continued cooperation the study depends, then such developments should only add to the value of this important study.

RWJ 10/05/02

# Index

Page numbers for photographs, boxes and figures are in italics.